To Ageless Margaret, with my best regards

"The truth at last! Dr. Ed Schneider knows more about increasing our healthspan than anyone I've interviewed over the years. In *The Longevity Quotient*, he's digested it all into the most comprehensive, least expensive, holistic health plan—which has the added benefit of inoculating us against anti-aging hype. And it goes down easier than the supplements you can now throw out!"

—**Gail Sheehy**, author of *New Passages* and *The Silent Passage*

"*The Longevity Quotient* gets it right! Longevity is about living better, not just longer. Dr. Edward Schneider's practical application of the latest science is a useful guide for maintaining vitality at any age."

—**John W. Rowe**, chairman and CEO of Aetna Inc. and author of *Successful Aging*

"With *The Longevity Quotient*, Dr. Schneider once again makes a significant contribution to the field of aging. Based on the most current and respected research, *The Longevity Quotient* is required reading for everyone who wants a long and healthy life."

—**Robert N. Butler**, MD, president and CEO of International Longevity Center–USA and author of *Why Survive? Being Old in America*

"The . . . wisdom Dr. Schneider prescribes in this book will keep us healthy and young at heart."

—**Betty Friedan**, author of *The Feminine Mystique* and *The Fountain of Age*

The Longevity Quotient

Calculate Your Odds of Aging Well—

and Take Steps Now to

Stay Youthful for Life

EDWARD L. SCHNEIDER, M.D.

Dean of the Leonard Davis School of Gerontology, University of Southern California

and Elizabeth Miles

RODALE

This book was previously published by Rodale Inc. as *AgeLess* (© 2003 by Edward L. Schneider, M.D.).

© 2003 by Edward L. Schneider, M.D.
Illustrations © 2003 by Karen Kuchar

All rights reserved. No part of this publication may be reproduced or transmitted in any form or by any means, electronic or mechanical, including photocopying, recording, or any other information storage and retrieval system, without the written permission of the publisher.

Printed in the United States of America
Rodale Inc. makes every effort to use acid-free ∞, recycled paper ♻.

"Recommended Total Daily Intake of Calcium" on page 55 is reprinted with permission from the National Academy of Sciences. Courtesy of the National Academics Press, Washington, D.C.

"Successful Versus Nonsuccessful Ways to Cope with Stress" on page 180 is adapted from *Aging Well* by George Vaillant. © 2002 by George E. Vaillant, M.D. Reprinted with permission from Little, Brown and Company, (Inc.).

Illustrations by Karen Kuchar
Book Design by Christina Gaugler

Library of Congress Cataloging-in-Publication Data

Schneider, Edward L.
    The longevity quotient : calculate your odds of aging well—and take steps now to stay youthful for life / Edward L. Schneider.
        p.   cm.
    Includes bibliographical references and index.
    ISBN 1–57954–986–1 paperback
    1. Longevity.   I. Title.
RA776.75.S333   2004
613'.0438—dc22   2004007528

Distributed to the book trade by St. Martin's Press

2   4   6   8   10   9   7   5   3   1   paperback

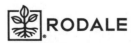

RODALE

WE **INSPIRE** AND **ENABLE** PEOPLE TO IMPROVE
THEIR LIVES AND THE WORLD AROUND THEM

FOR PRODUCTS & INFORMATION
www.**RODALESTORE**.com
www.**PREVENTION**.com

(800) 848-4735

This book is dedicated to the joys of my life, my wife Leah
and my children Samuel, Isaac, Clare, and Jakub.

Contents

Acknowledgments

I want to start by acknowledging my wonderful grandparents, Isadore and Minnie Soskin, for inspiring me to pursue a career serving older persons. Over the last three decades, this motivation has been rekindled by all the seniors whom I have met at my talks or during my encounters at the National Institute on Aging and the University of Southern California. My career in aging research was nourished by the great leaders in the field of aging, Nathan Shock, Robert Butler, and T. Franklin Williams. Colleagues who inspired me throughout my career include John W. Rowe, James Smith, Caleb Finch, Jack Guralnick, Mitchell Reff, Eric Stanbridge, Jacob Brody, Terry Fulmer, Gail Sheehy, Betty Friedan, and Warren Bennis. Here at USC, I have received strong support as Dean from President Steven Sample, Provosts Neil Pings and Lloyd Armstrong, and Vice Provosts Robert Biller, Sylvia Manning, Michael Diamond, Marty Levine, and Joe Hellige, as well as by the world-class faculty, staff, and students of the Leonard Davis School of Gerontology.

This book would not have occurred without the constant urging of my dear friends Keith Renken and Gale Bensussen. It could not have been written without the aid of the staff of the Andrus Gerontology Center, including Serena Sanker, Rhea Rebbe, Long-Hai Pham, Scott Gillies, Eun-Hae Kim, Stella Fu, and particularly Gitta Morris, who has been at my side for over 16 years as my executive assistant. And it might never have been published without the skills of Betsy Amster, who guided me through the world of commercial publishing and introduced me to the incredibly talented Elizabeth Miles.

I want to single out Rebecca Morris for working above and well beyond the call of duty to insure that all the references for the citations in the book were accurate, up-to-date and appropriate. Without her, we could never have delivered the book to the publishers on time and in great condition. I also wish to thank Ginny Faber and all the fine staff of Rodale whose editorial skills vastly improved the quality of this book.

It was important that the statements in this book be validated by experts in each field covered, and we were blessed with the great expertise of William Dement, Robert Sapolsky, Walter Willett, Kathy Smith, and Carrie Wiatt. I was also fortunate to have my caring physician and expert on General Internal Medicine, Dr. John Broadhead, review the manuscript and add his helpful insights. We also appreciate comments and suggestions received from Drs. Michael Holick, David Woodley, and Susan Love.

Last, but certainly not least, I want to thank my loving wife Leah and my wonderful children Samuel, Isaac, Clare, and Jakub for their patience and unwavering encouragement.

—Edward L. Schneider, M.D.

My thanks to the amazing AgeLess team—my coauthor Ed, whose humor, aplomb, and passion for our topic got me through many twists and turns in the road. The rare and lovely Rebecca Morris; your research savvy and attention to detail allowed me to stay happily lost in the words. Gitta Morris made everything work and everything a pleasure. Our agent Betsy Amster helped forge our partnership and keep the project on track with saintly patience and smart advice. At Rodale, thanks to Tami Booth for bringing the book into the fold; to Susan Berg, who nurtured the early seed; and to Ginny Faber, who bravely demanded our best when we were getting weary. And always, thanks to my friends and family for cheering me on when I'm writing and providing the reward when I'm not. You are my best reasons for living long and well.

—Elizabeth Miles

CHAPTER 1

AGELESS

As **THE DEAN** of the nation's only School of Gerontology, I am devoted to increasing health and vitality through aging research and education. For three decades, I've participated in a radical shift in our understanding of the aging process. While scientists once thought that the secret to longevity was to choose healthy grandparents who lived to a ripe old age—not an easy proposition—we now have the evidence to prove that it's not all in your genes. In fact, your daily actions and attitudes are the strongest influence on how well you age, via specific biochemical and neurological effects on your biological clock. This means that the ability to increase your health and longevity is in your hands.

Leading these advances was the landmark MacArthur Foundation Study of Successful Aging, a pivotal investigation that changed how we view the aging process. I was part of the MacArthur research team, which looked at data from the Swedish Twin Study. The study followed 20,000 identical and nonidentical twins, raised together and apart, for over 40 years—an ideal situation for studying genetic and environmental factors for health and disease. We specifically focused on how much genes and the environment each contributed to how well people aged.

The results were astounding. We found that while genes can play an important role in health during the early decades of life, from there on out (most of adulthood) your behaviors and lifestyle account for *a full 70 percent of how well you age.* In other words, genetic influences on your longevity diminish substantially as you move down life's path. Your own behaviors take their place.

The MacArthur study went on to identify the top habits of highly successful agers. As one example, we found that people who stayed the most mentally sharp exercised more, achieved higher levels of education, and had better self-efficacy—belief in one's ability to organize and execute actions to achieve specific goals. Similar blueprints emerged for the many aspects of aging—or more aptly, aging less.

AgeLess living is a comprehensive concept. Following from the MacArthur study and the wealth of other good research now available, I've grounded this book not just on a single theory of aging, destined to pass into history with the next trend, but on an integrated model that covers every aspect of your daily life that influences the aging process. From what you eat and how well you sleep to the type and length of your exercise routine, weight management issues, how you cope with stress, and your hormonal profile, you can acquire the AgeLess practices that will enable you to live longer with more zest and vitality. This book will show you how.

Take Control of Your Age

We all age differently. If you've ever been to a high school or college re-union, you've seen the proof up close. The prom king might look decades older than the calendar says, while the formerly mousy math whiz radiates youthful vitality and dances the night away. Though the chronological clock ticks at the same rate for all of us, everyone's bio-logical clock has its own speed. To a great extent, you can control that rate. Though you can't stop aging, as some people and products might claim, you *can* age less.

The essential part of ourselves, whether you call it soul, self, or spirit, is ageless. This ageless self enables us to identify with the youthful pro-tagonists in coming-of-age films and books because, internally, we feel eternally young. This book offers you tools to minimize the toll of time and maximize the correspondence between your ageless self and the face that meets the world. By adopting AgeLess principles, you can in-crease your vitality today, prevent or postpone the diseases of aging, and add healthy years to your time on earth.

Live Well to Age Well

The goal of an AgeLess lifestyle is a longer *healthspan,* my term for the healthy and active part of lifespan. Aging is a lifelong process: Soon after conception, as the human embryo grows, certain cells start to age and die. As our lives grow longer, so does the drama of age. At present, it is not possible to stop or reverse aging. If you're alive, you're getting older, and anyone who claims otherwise is misleading you. However, you *can* significantly slow the age-related processes that clog arteries and raise blood pressure, impair sugar metabolism, turn firm muscles to flab, sap energy, weaken and wrinkle the skin, and attack memory and mental functions. AgeLess habits can alter the course of countless biological reactions to help prevent many of the disorders and diseases associated with aging: heart disease, stroke, adult-onset diabetes, most cancers, disability, memory loss, and more. They can also address the myriad cosmetic concerns that mount with the years—weight gain, wrinkles, sagging flesh, and fading glow. In short, the way you live can largely determine your youthfulness today and how long and healthy your later life will be. An AgeLess lifestyle can optimize your chance of becoming a centenarian and still having plenty of juice left when you get there.

My own grandparents were AgeLess role models for me. Though I knew them for 40 years, I never saw these two dynamos grow old. Their joie de vivre communicated an agelessness that would one day become the elixir that I now offer to all of you. My grandmother lived life to the fullest throughout her eighties, doing her own housekeeping and shopping, cooking for her grandchildren, running out to have fun with her friends at the senior center, and still having time left over to volunteer at the local nursing home. My grandfather was equally active, managing his apartment building and playing vigorously with his grandchildren. He never lost his energy or gusto for life.

During my medical training, I didn't understand what the doctors meant when they discussed old age in a negative way. These vital, engaged, and energetic people were proof to me that aging didn't mean the inevitable decline that my medical teachers described. My grandparents inspired me to make the study of aging my life's work.

We live at a time of unprecedented opportunity to maximize our AgeLess potential. In the United States, average life expectancy at birth has increased from 49 years in 1900 to over 77 today. Most readers of this book will make it to age 85, and many of you have a good shot at celebrating your 100th birthday. But with current trends, half of our future 85-year-olds will need help with simple daily tasks due to age-related infirmities acquired along the way. Which will you be—independent, vigorous, and active, or needy, disabled, and sick? Now is the time to decide.

Healthspan Matters at Any Age

This is an all-ages book. If you don't think aging less is your concern yet, you're in good company. Ethel Percy Andrus, a dedicated educator a few decades ago, couldn't be bothered with aging or its negative stereotypes until she unexpectedly received her retirement notice from the Los Angeles Unified School District. One of the first women high school principals during the Depression and after, Ethel rejected the district's measly fixed $100 monthly pension and instead took a step that would transform the face of aging in America. Ethel cofounded AARP to lead the battle for the right of people of all ages to enjoy life to its peak potential.

AARP is now one of the largest and most powerful organizations in the world, 35 million members strong and regularly ranked the nation's leading lobbying group. Since Ethel Andrus was an educator committed to the empowering nature of knowledge, it was fitting that the AARP should decide to found a research center in her name to study the science of aging. They chose the University of Southern California as the site and invited the association's members to contribute to the center's construction and endowment. The response was astonishing. The state-of-the-art Ethel Percy Andrus Gerontology Center was built with contributions from more than *400,000 private citizens*, most of them retired, setting a world record for the most individual contributions toward the construction of a single nonreligious building.

Why such enthusiasm and generosity from people whom others assumed to be more interested in retirement than in new discoveries? My experience as a gerontologist shows that once you get to the so-called golden years, whether you find them to be golden or instead see rust spots everywhere and wish you could do it all over again, you realize just how important the length of your healthspan is. The idea of improving prospects for long, independent lives was so moving to these donors that they opened their hearts and wallets to help make it happen. They acted on what they knew firsthand to be a top priority for realizing their own dreams and desires: having the knowledge they needed to optimize their age potential. Though society didn't have a dream for them—or worse, expected them to be invisible—the spark of life in each was fanned by this woman's determination to make a difference to the core definition of longevity.

Le Troisième Age

The French have a wonderful term for the golden years: *le troisième age*, or the third age. After youth and middle age comes this time, which can be tough if you're unprepared but sweet if you've planned ahead. Age less today to make the third age your best life stage.

Today I head up the Ethel Percy Andrus Gerontology Center at The University of Southern California, where Ethel's legacy has inspired me to write this book to bring all the benefits of scientific knowledge about aging to people everywhere. Ethel, whose savings were wiped out by the Depression, once said, "What I have saved is lost, what I have spent is gone, but what I have given to other people is mine forever." Now, I would like to offer you the gift of a longer healthspan.

The benefits of aging less extend across the lifespan. If you're in your thirties or forties, you'll be glad to hear that now, the very time you start to get concerned about the first gray hairs, a "senior moment" memory lapse, or extra pounds you swear you didn't earn, can be the most effective moment to adopt strategies for aging less. Those of you in your fifties and sixties can see rapid improvements to health and vitality by making those changes to arrest or slow many of the conditions associated with age. To seniors, I offer a rejuvenating program that's easy and affordable so your golden years can live up to your dreams. For readers in your twenties, remember that controlling your healthspan is as important as making good choices for your career, personal relationships, and your portfolio. Just as financial experts advise that you begin planning for retirement as soon as you finish college, your investment in longevity today can yield great benefits far into the future.

Many Americans alive today have the opportunity to see a century of good living *if* they start now. You can use our Longevity Quotient Plan to lengthen your healthspan, and the earlier you start the greater improvement you can make. So, no matter what your current age or genetic background, age less by living well each day to promote:

⑥ Longer healthspan
⑥ Optimal heart health, bone mass, and digestion
⑥ Energy, stamina, and strength

⑥ Youthful appearance and healthy body weight
⑥ Better cognition and memory
⑥ Improved mood and optimism
⑥ Satisfying sex
⑥ Money saved on health care and antiaging products
⑥ Fewer sick days
⑥ Sound sleep
⑥ Clear vision
⑥ Enhanced performance
⑥ A life-embracing mind-set
⑥ Independence and vitality far into the future

What would you add to this list? How do you envision your third age? Who are the role models in your life who seem to transcend aging? Use these questions as your compass and begin to chart your AgeLess healthspan today.

Discover Your Longevity Quotient—and Change It

Will you be playing tennis on your 85th birthday or struggling to get out of a chair at 60? Should you expect your energy and sex drive to fizzle by age 45 or will you hit middle age with body and mind in their prime?

To help you measure your healthspan—*and change it*—I've developed a measurement I call the longevity quotient (LQ). You're probably already familiar with this sort of assessment in the form of the intelligence quotient (IQ) test, which was introduced by Dr. William Louis Stern in 1912 to predict how an individual will perform in comparison to the population on various cognitive tasks. Likewise, I've developed my LQ quizzes to size up your habits to help assess the length and quality of your healthspan in six key areas.

The Six-Point LQ Plan to Increase Your Healthspan

The habits that can help you age less fall into six categories.

1. Nutrition
2. Exercise
3. Weight management
4. Sleep
5. Engagement with life
6. Hormone replacement

The LQ quizzes provided in the upcoming chapters can help you to see where you're on track for a long, vigorous life and where you have room to improve. If you score 100 percent on all the quizzes, congratulations! Hand this book to someone who can use it. For the rest of you (and that's most of us), a true assessment of your current situation is critical to prioritizing your personal longevity plan, so be honest with yourself: Stick with what *is* rather than what you wish would be. Use photocopies of the quizzes if you're reluctant to commit your secrets to these pages. If you prefer, you can complete the LQ quizzes online at www.longevityquotient.com. These interactive versions handle all the calculations for you.

As they say on the radio when they try out the emergency broadcast system, the LQ is "only a test." The results don't cast your future in stone; in fact, quite the opposite. With these tests and the six-point LQ plan, you can take control of your future—perhaps for the first time—and decide for yourself how to increase your healthspan. Seeing is believing, and your LQ score can provide the framework you need to start aging less today.

As you total up your LQ in each area, focus on the big picture. How do you feel about your score? Is it surprising? Reassuring? Disconcerting? First, remember that this number is designed to help you chart your course; it's not a judgment of your worth, intent, or intelligence. More importantly, whether the number you see on the page is high, low, or in between, the key fact is that *your longevity quotient can change* for the better, if you begin implementing the LQ plan. And *your longevity quotient is cumulative;* every day you spend following your LQ plan is money in the bank. You are investing in your present and future—so the sooner you start, the higher your lifelong LQ will be.

Heed the New Rules of Aging Less

I've spent 30 years fielding questions about how to live a long and healthy life. As befits my Jewish heritage, I've freely dispensed solicited and unsolicited advice to just about anyone who has asked. What's amazing is how much the answers have changed over the course of my career.

As science has revolutionized so many aspects of our lives, it's also changed the face of aging. Since the 1960s, the baby boom generation has influenced every aspect of our society—how we work, play, and maintain our health and well-being. Now, as this dynamic group prepares to enter its third age, its members are enthusiastically looking for ways to stay youthful, but often without the latest information.

The majority of people I meet are following old, outdated rules. In this book, I lay out the New Rules of aging less—cutting-edge knowledge based on the newest, most credible research that will help you maximize your LQ.

Why the Old Rules No Longer Apply

In many cases, factors that we thought were important for successful aging have been proven wrong by newer and often better-controlled studies. Sometimes there was no solid scientific basis to begin with—the federal government's Food Guide Pyramid, for example. Other old rules sprang from popular misconceptions, such as the idea that you should be as thin as you possibly can. The old rules had too many of the 55 percent of Americans officially considered overweight, unhappily dieting. Now we know that a few extra pounds can save your life; in fact for many of us, stepping off the diet treadmill can help preserve our health, wealth, and sanity.

Many of the old rules were based on what are called observational studies, in which researchers look at such health behaviors as eating habits or exercise in groups of individuals and correlate them with specific diseases they may acquire over time. If the results of one of these studies showed that those in the group who exercised more had fewer heart attacks, we could conclude that exercise prevents heart disease. Some large-scale, long-term observational studies that you might have heard of include the Nurses' Health Study, the Health Professionals' Follow-Up Study, and the Framingham Heart Study. Some very important findings have come out of these. For instance, the Framingham Heart Study was the first to link elevated cholesterol, inactivity, and smoking to heart disease.

While the findings from observational studies can seem remarkable, some of those termed breakthroughs have not stood up to the next level of scientific scrutiny. Beta-carotene is a case in point. Initial observational studies suggested that individuals who consumed more beta-carotene in their diets had a significantly lower risk of heart disease. Predictably, plenty of people started taking beta-carotene supplements in hopes of gaining the protection the study found. Then came the more rigorous randomized, placebo-controlled, double-blinded clinical studies that can definitively examine cause and effect. This gold standard for research involves randomly placing participants into two groups who get either a supplement or a placebo, and neither doctor nor patient knows who's getting what until the study is completed. Such controlled studies of beta-carotene supplements failed to show any beneficial effects, and some even hinted at a possible increase in the risk of cancer. There goes the old rule.

The problem with observational studies is that certain behaviors can go together and there's no way to know which one caused the effect. Look at the case of vitamin E. In two very large studies of men and women conducted by the Harvard School of Public Health, the Nurses' Health Study and the Health Professionals' Follow-Up Study, participants who took vitamin E supplements had less heart disease than those who didn't. However, those who took these supplements also had better health habits overall, including eating right, exercising, watching their weight, and not smoking. More recent randomized, placebo-controlled, double-blinded studies show no relationship between taking vitamin E supplements and the risk of getting heart disease. Therefore, in the observational studies, it was probably the good health habits, not the vitamin pills, that accounted for the supplement takers' health advantage.

We're seeing a similar pattern among women who take estrogen. While early observational studies reported a lower risk of heart disease in women on hormone replacement therapy, the National Institutes of Health–sponsored Women's Health Initiative study of estrogen and progestin was recently stopped three years earlier than planned because the initial results so clearly showed that hormone replacement did not provide protection, and, in fact, caused slightly more harm than good.

The Old Rules Were Hard to Follow

I remember exhorting people seeking the keys to aging less to work hard at their goals. Run 5 miles a day! Peel off those extra pounds! Slash the fat in your diet! Avoid stress whenever you can!

Giving this advice was easy. What was hard was finding anyone who could stick with the program. We'd set the bar too high.

It was a great relief when scientific studies started to show that we could relax these rigid rules. Yes, vigorous exercise is great, but just getting off the couch will improve your health and longevity. While I'd love to see you eat at least five servings of vegetables and fruits each day, getting in even one additional portion can reduce your heart disease and cancer risk. And you definitely don't want to trim all the fat from your diet; some fats are longevity boosters! As for those 10 pounds you think you have to lose, hold on. Being too thin can be bad for your healthspan, and excessive weight loss and fad diets can actually age the body.

In fact, to maximize healthspan, one of the best things you can do is take it easy. Take breaks from the frantic pace of overscheduling or feeling that you can never do enough. Work less and spend more time getting plenty of sleep and investing in relationships. Toss out that medicine chest full of dietary supplements and focus on a few nutrition basics. Delete "no pain, no gain" from your vocabulary and find an exercise routine that feels natural and fun. Pain can cause premature aging; the New Rules help you retain youthfulness while being nice to yourself.

Information Overload

A staggering amount of health information is available to the average consumer. Conflicting study results reported by the media, not to mention advertising claims, have most Americans feeling overwhelmed and frustrated. If you take every new finding as gospel, you'll stay confused forever.

As a modern-day consumer, you've doubtlessly come across advertisements for coenzyme Q_{10}, ginkgo biloba, high-protein diets, human growth hormone, and many more elixirs of the fountain of youth. You've read the amazing claims that these products will keep your muscles firm and your skin wrinkle-free. Even sophisticated consumers might be fooled into signing up for a "colonic cleansing" that promises to remove all impurities from the body and restore its natural balance (an enema in disguise), popping the latest "natural" diet pill (usually some sort of stimulant), or taking DHEA in hopes of stopping age in its tracks (it doesn't). In the face of this information overload, how do you sift the chaff from the wheat?

The Long View of Longevity

There has never been so much interest in longevity and age as there is today nor so many people eager to offer their personal take on the topic. Many books on aging are written by authors from other disciplines, from veterinarians to dentists, nutritionists to personal trainers. While I welcome this wide discussion, it's discouraging to see innocent people try ineffective, sometimes dangerous ways to restore their youth.

Aging well is my life's work. I've dedicated my professional career to scientific research and education on the aging process. Like most of you, during my youth I didn't give much thought to growing old. I was far more concerned with winning sailboat races and skiing black diamond trails. Still, as a doctor, I was fascinated by the riddle of age. Why, after spending all that time acquiring so much knowledge and experience, do we begin the inevitable path toward our demise?

After med school and residency, I began my work as a researcher at the University of California, San Francisco, looking at how cells age. Later, I joined the newly born National Institute on Aging (part of the federal government's National Institutes of Health), where as a molecular biologist, I examined how aging cells responded to environmental damage. After working with my staff to create new national programs to discover the causes of Alzheimer's disease and encourage clinical research on aging, I ended up the Institute's deputy director. Entrusted with giving away hundreds of millions of dollars in federal grants related to aging, I saw proposals cross my desk when the studies were just gleams in the scientists' eyes. It was an exciting vantage point from which to watch the development of aging research around the world.

I am equally excited today, as the Dean of the Leonard Davis School of Gerontology at the University of Southern California, where our faculty pursues up-to-the-minute social, psychological, and policy research as well as biomedical investigations of aging. With this perspective that my experience provides, you can understand why I get upset when people make misleading claims or offer irresponsible advice about aging—and how I sympathize with the consumer's feelings of confusion and overload. In my many years in the field, I've seen estrogen go in and out of favor several times. I've witnessed the melatonin miracle and the DHEA revolution and then watched them disappear. I participated in early studies and have followed the evidence for decades. I've watched many books report the latest fads only to see their recommendations refuted with the next scientific finding and stood by while so-called "miracle" pills came and went.

Through it all, I have sorted through the findings to select only the best, most valid studies. In this book, I have distilled them into concise recommendations for you. I waited a long time to write this book because the science of aging less through lifestyle choices wasn't yet ready for prime time. Now, at last, it is, and I've written these New Rules to make optimizing healthspan easy for everyone.

Sound Medical Research: Beyond the Breakthroughs

So where do the findings behind the New Rules come from? They came from thousands of studies published in the top peer-reviewed journals. I've traced the science of each rule back through its history and accounted for the full balance of evidence—not the latest "breakthrough." The New Rules are exciting because they break the old rules and make extending your healthspan easier than ever before. And because they take the long view, the New Rules will also serve you well far into the future. (Visit www.longevityquotient.com for updates.)

As much as possible, the New Rules are based on the gold standard for research: randomized, double-blinded, placebo-controlled studies. Obviously, this design works best for pills. The best behavior-based studies compare one behavior—for example, of exercise—with another health behavior like taking supplements or participating in an educational group.

I've based each New Rule on the preponderance of evidence from the strongest, best-designed studies conducted by leading experts on the issue. The references in the back of the book give you just a sampling of this work. If you take an interest, by all means head for the library or to the Internet to see the data at its source. If not, don't worry. I've done the hard work for you, and the New Rules translate complex research into simple lifestyle measures.

It's important to note that the New Rules are based on the very best science, while many antiaging claims don't meet even minimal scientific standards. I've attended plenty of talks in which the speaker claims "I know it works and so do those people who've used it," effectively dismissing the need for rigorous scientific studies. No matter how many glowing testimonials you hear, even from sources you respect, don't be taken in by anecdotal evidence! Even the most intelligent individual can experience a short-term placebo effect from any given treatment; the novelty and heightened expectation of trying something new can buoy your feeling of well-being.

Keeping an Open Mind: Considering Alternatives and Options

In addition to better research, we have taken more alternative routes to aging less than ever before. As a doctor and patient alike, I've always been open to new approaches to health. I've traveled in China, studying acupuncture and other aspects of traditional Chinese medicine and have been involved in studies of Chinese herbal remedies. For the arthritis I acquired from various skiing mishaps described in embarrassing detail in chapter 3, I take the complementary remedy glucosamine and chondroitin sulfate three times a day. Approximately half of arthritis patients who take this preparation get some pain relief, and I'm among them. Studies show that echinacea can be effective in improving immune function, and saw palmetto can delay prostate enlargement.

However, many complementary remedies have not lived up to all their claims, including ginseng and ginkgo biloba. Others, such as ephedra, are frankly dangerous. Some, including colonic cleansing and certain herbal concoctions, are disagreeable in addition to being useless for health or aging less.

The New Rules encompass a wide variety of approaches to staying youthful, from meditation to tai chi, estrogen alternatives, and a nutritional plan that draws on nature's best.

Easy, Enjoyable, Affordable, and Safe: Gain without Pain

I learned early in my medical career that you can be the cleverest doctor in the world in diagnosing a patient's ailments, but you haven't helped until you provide a course of action that he or she can actually follow. That's why I keep the New Rules easy for everyone to achieve. Are you "allergic" to exercise? Try the "I-Don't-Have-Time-to-Exercise" program in chapter 3, specially designed for extremely busy or workout-averse people. Is your budget too tight to buy lots of supplements? You don't have to. I'll tell you which few are important to your healthspan and how, when, and why you need to take them. Too tired to read a treatise on how to get more youth-boosting sleep? Skip to the Top 10 Tips in chapter 5. And if you associate healthy eating with tasteless food and deprivation, check out our yummy snack in chapter 2—dark chocolate-covered walnuts.

You can spend a fortune on remedies to improve your health and longevity. When I visited a health food store in Berkeley, California, and asked for supplements to improve my health and longevity, they gave me a list that added up to over $600 for a 1- to 2-month supply. By contrast, the LQ plan should cost you $10 or less each month for the select supplements I recommend.

Though scientific information can get complicated, the New Rules keep the process simple and a source of daily pleasure. Just follow the AgeLess plan, and you'll have more vitality today and plenty of time to achieve your dreams.

CHAPTER 2

NUTRITION

OLD NUTRITION RULE	NEW NUTRITION RULE
Take a daily multivitamin as one-stop nutrition insurance.	**#1.** Toss your multivitamin.
Fruits and vegetables are supporting players.	**#2.** Eat five or more servings of fruits and vegetables a day.
Fats are bad for you.	**#3.** Don't cut back on fats—just choose the right ones.
Eat the diet recommended by the USDA Food Guide Pyramid.	**#4.** Follow the AgeLess Nutrition Pyramid.
Ward off age by swallowing a kitchen sink's worth of dietary supplements.	**#5.** Take only the supplements you need: calcium, vitamin D, folic acid, and if you're over 55 or a vegan, vitamin B_{12}.

I WAS VISITING MY MOTHER in the nursing home when I got the now familiar question. Patricia, one of the nurse's aides taking care of Mom, pulled me aside for a private chat.

Because she saw the consequences of aging every day, Patricia, age 45, considered her health a top priority. She told me that she was spending more than $175 a month on dietary supplements. "I know they're supposed to be an investment in my future," she confided, "but taking all these pills every day is draining my bank account. What should I do?"

Like many people, Patricia had heeded every promotion put out by the supplement industry. Eager to reap the benefits promised for each pill, she had tried just about everything. Her medicine cabinet contained a multivitamin, a vitamin B-complex pill, and an antioxidant mix, along with separate bottles of vitamins A, C, D, and E, beta carotene, calcium, magnesium, chromium, zinc, choline, creatine, ginseng, ginkgo biloba, omega-3 fatty acids, blue-green algae, St. John's wort, shark cartilage, royal jelly, coenzyme Q_{10}, phytoestrogens, DHEA, melatonin, echinacea, lutein, flaxseed oil, MSM, grapeseed oil, and linoleic acid.

I told Patricia to get back to basics: Forget the plethora of pills and heed proven science. I pointed out that if she put that $175 a month in a retirement account instead of spending it on substances of no use to her healthspan, she could simplify her life now and celebrate her 70th birthday with an extra $93,000 in the bank.

Your diet is critically important to your health—but I bet some of my nutrition advice surprises you. When I told Patricia to toss out her multivitamins, I meant it. The real longevity power of nutrients is hidden in foods—the same ones you shop for at your supermarket.

Patricia now spends less than $10 a month on dietary supplements and enjoys good health and a new appreciation for food. You can, too. This chapter will teach you how to eat your way to a longer, more delicious life.

WHAT'S YOUR LONGEVITY QUOTIENT?

Nutrition

Take the following quiz to assess the effects of your eating habits on your healthspan. Add up the LQ points you earn in each area and enter the total in the "Your LQ Points" column. Be sure not to exceed the maximum score allowed for each item. For example, your fruit and vegetable score tops out at 50, even if you eat more than five servings a day. If you eat two portions of fruits and two portions of vegetables each day, you would write down "40" on the line under "Your LQ Points" (4 × 10 points = 40 points). If you eat 6 portions, even though this is terrific, you still put only "50" in the column.

	Your LQ Points	Max LQ Points
Fruits and Vegetables		
10 points: For each portion of fruits and vegetables you eat each day (1 portion = ½ cup)	___	**50**

	Your LQ Points	Max LQ Points

Nuts

1 point: For each portion (1 ounce) of nuts you eat each week   ____   **5**

Fish

2½ points: For each serving of fish you eat each week   ____   **5**

Calcium

5 points: For each 500-milligram calcium supplement you
        take each day

2½ points: For each cup of milk or yogurt you consume
        each day

1 point: For each multivitamin tablet you take each day that
        contains 160 milligrams of calcium

1 point: For eating lots of vegetables, soy products, or both   ____   **10**

Vitamin D

If you are 65 and older:

1 point: For each 5 minutes you spend each week outdoors
        in sunshine without sunscreen and with face, arms,
        and hands exposed

1 point: For each hour you spend each week outdoors in sunshine
        with sunscreen and with face, arms, and hands exposed

If you are 21 to 64:

4 points: For each 5 minutes you spend each week outdoors
        in sunshine without sunscreen and with face, arms,
        and hands exposed

4 points: For each hour you spend each week outdoors in
        sunshine with sunscreen and with face, arms, and
        hands exposed

All ages:

8 points: If you take daily supplements containing
        1,000 IU vitamin D

3 points: If you take a daily multivitamin or separate
        supplement containing 400 IU vitamin D

1 point: For each glass of vitamin D-enriched milk you   ____   **8**
        drink per day

	Your LQ Points	Max LQ Points

Folate

    8 points: For each 800-microgram (or more) folic acid
             supplement you take each day

    4 points: For each 400-microgram folic acid supplement
             you take each day

    4 points: If you take a multivitamin

| 1 point: For each serving of bread, cereal, or other grain you eat each day | ____ | 8 |

Red Meat

    How often do you eat red meat (beef, pork, lamb, including cold cuts, hot dogs, hamburgers, sausage, and so forth)?

    3 points: Once a week or less

    2 points: Two times a week

    1 point: Three or four times a week

| 0 points: Five times a week or more | ____ | 3 |

Whole Grains and Legumes

| 2 points: For each portion of whole grains or legumes you eat per day | ____ | 4 |

Fats

    What do you usually cook with?

    3 points: Olive or canola oil

    2 points: Vegetable or corn oil

| 0 points: Butter, margarine, shortening, or lard | ____ | 3 |

Water

| 1 point: For each glass of fluid you drink each day (except for coffee, tea, soft drinks, and alcohol) | ____ | 4 |

| **Total** | ____ | **100** |

What does your nutrition LQ forecast for your future? Find your score in the following list to read my diagnosis:

Total LQ Score	The Dean's Diagnosis
91–100	You're a nutritional champ! Stick to your smart habits but read this chapter for some surprise pointers.
81–90	You're on track, but there's room for improvement. Some fine-tuning of your diet will better protect you against the diseases of aging.
71–80	Wake-up call: You're not eating to optimize your healthspan. It's time to make some changes.
61–70	Danger zone! Your dietary choices are jeopardizing your healthspan. You need to make a serious commitment to change.
60 or below	Disaster zone. You're at great risk for the diseases and disorders of aging and need to overhaul your eating habits from the ground up.

Whatever your score, take heart! Eating for a long, healthy life is a pleasure.

Your Age Is What You Eat

Even small improvements to your diet can be beneficial. You can help prevent colon cancer, for instance, with just one more serving of a fruit or vegetable per day. One study found that people who averaged 1½ daily servings of fruits and vegetables were 65 percent more likely to develop colon cancer than those who upped their consumption to just 2½ servings per day. That's a lot of protection for one portion of veggies or fruit!

Nutrition has a cumulative effect on the aging process. The right foods are natural pharmaceuticals in that they support healthy bio-chemical reactions, cell division, and cardiovascular function, and the powerful benefits accrue over time. Even better, AgeLess eating can im-prove your energy and appearance right now. Every day that you feed yourself well helps your healthspan, so it's never too early or too late to start.

You may balk at the idea of eating right if you remember the health food movement of the 1960s and 1970s—days of brewer's yeast and sprouts—or suffered the austere restrictions of the first very low fat diets for heart disease. Put these ghosts behind you! We've finally figured out that eating well can taste great. Yes, you can gracefully weather the years

Nutrition

Eat according to the New Nutrition Rules to help protect against and treat these diseases and conditions:

- Heart disease
- Stroke
- Cancer (many types)
- Diabetes
- Arthritis
- Diverticulitis and other digestive disease
- Hip and spinal fractures
- Cataracts
- Macular degeneration

An AgeLess diet can also boost your energy, enhance your immunity, and improve your appearance.

---

without eating strange or dull foods, and, no, you don't have to say goodbye to all fat forever. AgeLess eating boils down to this: Most of your nutrition should come from food, with a few supplements to close the gap in longevity-critical nutrients too hard to get enough of from your diet.

NEW NUTRITION RULE #1:
TOSS YOUR MULTIVITAMIN

Decades ago, as research began to reveal the importance of nutrition to health, the government came up with the recommended dietary allowances (RDAs)—the minimum daily intake to prevent deficiency in a healthy population (as opposed to an individual)—for vitamins, selected minerals, and other nutrients. The RDA numbers you find on food labels today are the targets that most people aim for. But don't be confused: There's no evidence that the RDAs, which are calculated strictly to keep you out of the danger zone, can optimize your healthspan and vitality! In fact, there's plenty of evidence to the contrary.

The word *vitamin* comes from the Greek *vita,* or life, and it describes any organic compound of carbon, hydrogen, and oxygen essential to human health that cannot be manufactured by your body. Researchers began identifying vitamins in the early 1900s, and with the discovery of vitamin C finally cleared up a medical mystery that dated back as far as 1500 B.C.—why did sailors on long voyages without fresh fruits and vegetables develop the potentially fatal disease called scurvy? Scientists knew that adding citrus fruit to sailors' diets prevented the disease, and they eventually figured out that the active ingredient was ascorbic acid—that is, vitamin C.

To determine the RDA for vitamin C, researchers experimented with a group of medical students (who have always been popular guinea pigs), giving them different amounts until they hit on just the dose—60 milligrams—to prevent scurvy. We've been stuck with that amount ever since.

Meanwhile, many studies have found that consuming more than the RDA of vitamin C can protect against heart disease, stroke, certain cancers, cataracts, and perhaps even the common cold—conditions that affect your healthspan. So the first step to AgeLess nutrition is to go beyond the RDAs.

Recognizing the limitations of the RDAs, the federal government has recently issued a new set of recommendations called dietary reference intakes (DRIs). These represent the levels of vitamins, minerals, and other nutrients believed to maximize health and prevent disease. The DRIs are divided by age and gender with special guidelines for pregnant and lactating women.

Our Supplement-Popping Society

It wasn't so long ago that mothers everywhere exhorted their children to eat right. These days, plenty of us are too busy swallowing supplements and chugging fortified drinks to pay attention to what's on anyone's plate—our children's or our own. But guess what? Most of the latest research points to the considerable advantages that food has over pills to improve health and longevity. Mom was right, and she still is.

Food contains powerful life-extending chemicals, such as antioxidants (vitamins C and E, and other compounds such as flavonoids and carotenoids), that work to optimize health and prevent premature cel-

What to Expect When . . .

Here are some of the signposts you might encounter in your eating patterns and nutritional needs as time goes by.

- **Twenties:** You feel fine no matter what you eat. Don't be fooled; youthful stamina and resilience can mask bad eating habits. Now is the time to develop good eating habits that can preserve your verve for a long time to come.

- **Thirties:** Suddenly, you're surprised to discover (and likely will try to ignore) a correlation between your eating habits and how you feel. You may become aware of your digestion for the first time. Bone strength and density peak and begin to decline during this decade, making it critical to get enough calcium and vitamin D. Adopt the New Rules recommendations to feel much better today while you protect your future healthspan.

- **Forties:** You're middle-aged. You need to fight back. Nutrition is your ace in the hole! Fortunately, the good eating habits you establish now are likely to stand you in good stead for the rest of your life.

- **Fifties and sixties:** As your stomach acid declines, so does your ability to absorb vitamin B_{12}. That's why age 55 is the time to start taking a B_{12} supplement.

- **Seventies:** Your thirst and fluid regulation mechanisms start to lose force, requiring an extra effort to drink enough water whether you think you want it or not. Your taste receptivity may also start to wane so that you can't rely on hunger to spur you to eat what you need. Nutrition may become more a conscious choice than a natural instinct.

- **Eighties and upward:** Time to put AgeLess eating on your must-do daily list. For many seniors, the day they stop eating is the day they start to die.

lular aging. After exercise, these naturally occurring chemicals may be the most important contributors to a long, vital life.

The processed and packaged foods that dominate the current American diet, however, have been stripped of valuable nutrients that naturally occur in whole, unprocessed foods. A quarter of the population pops multivitamins, hoping to compensate for the shortfall. Ironically, the same manufacturers who process away vital nutrients often fortify their nutritionally depleted foods with chemical isolates and imply in their advertisements and claims that these products improve upon nature.

Whether or not they take pills, most Americans consume a vast array of manufactured supplements, mixed into foods from breakfast cereal to energy bars, even café lattes—yet only about one in five gets the recommended five daily servings of vegetables and fruits.

Yet, a large body of scientific evidence shows that getting your vitamins from food is far preferable to obtaining them from supplements.

The Problem with Multivitamins

Let's look at America's favorite pill, the multivitamin. Most provide only the RDAs, and some don't even do that. At the time of this writing, for instance, one popular brand supplies only 16 percent of the RDA for calcium, a very important mineral. Daily multivitamins don't contain enough vitamin D or folic acid either. If we rely on multivitamins to fill in the gaps in our diets, we can end up with a sense of nutritional security that's utterly false.

Furthermore, many multivitamins contain the potent oxidants iron and copper, which may speed cellular aging and contribute to the development of arterial plaque. Your goal is to get more *anti*oxidants, not oxidants! While some menstruating or pregnant women and people with iron-deficient anemia may be correctly advised by their doctors to take iron supplements, there's no reason for healthy men, postmenopausal women, or younger women with adequate iron intake to expose themselves to additional oxidative substances—like the 18 milligrams of iron in the popular multivitamin tablet we just mentioned.

Another problem with multivitamins is all the other stuff that manufacturers throw in as added bait for you to buy them, from plant extracts, such as ginseng, with no known biological effects, to untested, potentially harmful additions like the so-called fat-burner, chromium picolinate. To make matters worse, the supplement industry remains largely unregulated for either the quality or quantity of its ingredients. Therefore, that pill you are taking, for example, may contain less than the label professes—or more, including contaminants.

I've distilled the full spectrum of good scientific research into the Age-Less Rules for daily nutrient intake. The table "Multivitamins versus Age-Less Recommendations" on page 24 provides a look at how some popular multivitamins stack up to these AgeLess requirements, which are based on the latest scientific research.

Multivitamins versus AgeLess Recommendations

This table shows the discrepancies between some popular multivitamins and the AgeLess recommendations.

	Vitamin B$_{12}$	Folic Acid	Vitamin C	Vitamin D
Multivitamin Centrum	6 mcg	400 mcg	60 mg	400 IU
Centrum Silver	25 mcg	400 mcg	60 mg	400 IU
Theragram-M Advanced Formula	12 mcg	400 mcg	90 mg	400 IU
Geritol Complete	6.7 mcg	380 mcg	57 mg	400 IU
One-A-Day Maximum	6 mcg	400 mcg	60 mg	400 IU
One-A-Day 50-Plus Formula	30 mcg	400 mcg	120 mg	400 IU
AgeLess Recommendations	**1,000 mcg over age 55**	**800 mcg from food and supplements**	**250 mg from food**	**1,000 IU from sun exposure, food, and supplements**

The Problem with Supplements

Besides the limitations of multivitamins is the more pressing problem of efficacy: Some nutrients that are good for your health when you eat them in food are of little use or even bad for you when you take them in chemically purified supplement form. An example is beta-carotene, which achieved great popularity as a supplement after studies showed that people with the highest blood beta-carotene levels had lower risks of heart disease and cancer. Then controlled studies showed that beta-carotene in supplement form does *not* protect against heart disease— and, if you smoke, taking beta-carotene supplements may actually *increase* your risk of cancer! How can science explain this contradiction?

The answer probably lies in the complex interactions of the many different chemicals that are found in foods. For instance, carrots contain beta-carotene (that's what makes them orange), but they also contain many other carotenoids such as alpha-carotene, cryptoxanthin, lutein, zeaxanthin, and lycopene. So it may be another carotenoid or a partic-

Vitamin E	Calcium	Iron	Copper
30 IU	162 mg	18 mg	2 mg
45 IU	200 mg	0 mg	2 mg
60 IU	40 mg	9 mg	2 mg
30 IU	148 mg	16 mg	1.8 mg
30 IU	162 mg	18 mg	2 mg
60 IU	120 mg	0 mg	2 mg
As much as possible from food (supplements optional)	1,000 to 1,500 mg from food and supplements	0* (food only)	0 (food only)

*Menstruating or pregnant women who do not get sufficient iron in their diets may require supplemental iron.

Data as of November 2002

ular combination that provides protection from heart disease and stroke.

This is an important lesson. We can't extrapolate from the results of studies involving food consumption of naturally occurring biochemicals to taking concentrations of a single, specific chemical. I hope you'll take a moment right now to go toss your beta-carotene supplements in the trash.

Perhaps the most controversial supplement is vitamin C. There's little question that fruits and vegetables high in vitamin C protect against heart disease, cancer, and cataracts. There is very little scientific evidence, however, that taking supplemental vitamin C offers the same protection. At this point, only dietary vitamin C is proven to promote good health.

Also consider the case of vitamin E. There was a time when "E" seemed to stand for "essential," and most health experts, myself included, recommended taking it to help protect against heart disease, Alzheimer's disease, and perhaps cellular aging itself.

A lot of the initial enthusiasm for vitamin E was based on findings of the Harvard Nurses' Health Study and the Health Professionals' Follow-Up Study, both reported in the *New England Journal of Medicine* in 1993. The Nurses' Health Study, an observational study, tracked the nutritional intake of 85,000 nurses for eight years and found that those who took supplemental vitamin E had the lowest risk of heart disease. A similar result came from 39,000 men participating in the Health Professionals' Follow-Up Study. Very large doses of vitamin E also appeared to slow down the progression of Alzheimer's disease. Since it was impossible to get adequate amounts through diet alone (100 to 400 milligrams a day) and there appeared to be no downside to supplementation, doctors said yes, and vitamin E sales soared.

But when supplemental vitamin E was subjected to double-blinded, placebo-controlled trials, pills alone proved to have no protective effect against heart disease. The researchers concluded that the health-conscious volunteers who took vitamin E supplements in the original studies might have been folks who exercised regularly, watched their waistlines, didn't smoke, and had other good health habits—and it may have been these practices, not supplemental vitamin E, that kept them well. On the other hand, we have good evidence that when eaten in food, vitamin E is good for you. These results suggest that supplements somehow miss the mark.

At a time when "more is better" sums up the general attitude toward nutritional supplementation, the New Rules call for caution. Vitamin E, for instance, acts as a blood thinner, and taking it in large doses can increase the risk of hemorrhagic stroke. In a large-scale study of 29,000 smokers, participants were given supplements of beta-carotene, vitamin E, or a placebo and followed for five to eight years. The results were not only surprising—they were a serious warning. Those taking the vitamin E had no reduction in their risk of lung cancer but showed an increased risk of hemorrhagic stroke, while those taking beta-carotene had an increased risk of lung cancer.

All that said, certain important nutrients are just too hard to get from food, and for these few vitamins and one mineral, I recommend taking separate supplements at my prescribed dose (not the government's RDAs). It's a little more complicated than grabbing a multivitamin, but the benefits are worth it. I'll cover these select supplements in New Rule #5.

NEW NUTRITION RULE #2:
EAT FIVE OR MORE SERVINGS
OF FRUITS AND VEGETABLES A DAY

Only 12 to 32 percent of Americans eat the recommended five daily servings of vegetables and fruits, depending upon which survey you read. One of the good ones, by the Centers for Disease Control and Prevention, canvassed 32,000 adults in 16 states and found that only 23 percent—fewer than one in four—got their daily five. This is a major problem for our healthspans, since diets rich in fruits and vegetables have consistently been found to help protect against heart disease and cancer, our leading causes of death, as well as stroke, diabetes, cataracts, macular degeneration, and diverticulitis. In a country where fresh produce packs the supermarkets all year round and everyone claims to be health- and weight-conscious, this gap is unconscionable.

If you make one change in your diet for a longer, better life, enjoying five or more daily servings of vegetables and fruits is the thing to do. In a society in which processed, packaged, and fast foods prevail and white flour, meat, sugar, and fat are the main ingredients of many a meal, this means going slightly against the grain. But make the effort. We are only beginning to truly grasp the power of plant foods, especially fruits and vegetables. Scientists are dissecting these natural wonders to discover healthful compounds we'd never even dreamed of. From antioxidants such as flavonoids and carotenoids to other vitamins, minerals, and fiber, fruits and vegetables offer a pharmacopoeia of health-enhancing substances.

The American Heart Association, the American Cancer Society, and the National Institutes of Health all recommend that Americans eat five to nine portions of fruits and vegetables a day. "What's a portion?" you may ask. Here's the answer.

Fruit

One portion equals:
- Medium-size apple, pear, banana, kiwifruit, orange
- ½ cup canned, chopped, cooked, or sectioned fruit
- 6 ounces fruit juice
- ¼ cup dried fruit

Vegetables

One portion equals:
- 1 cup raw green leafy vegetables
- ½ cup all other vegetables
- 6 ounces vegetable juice or soup

A Harvard study tracking more than 120,000 men and women for eight to fourteen years found that each additional daily serving of vegetables or fruits the participants consumed reduced their risk of coronary heart disease by 4 percent—so have another apple!

The Antioxidant Edge

Among the AgeLess benefits you'll find in fruits and vegetables are antioxidants—important longevity allies. Oxygen is necessary to life, but the chemical reaction that follows taking a big breath of air can also age your body. During the process of respiration, oxygen is converted into highly reactive biochemicals called free radicals. These free radicals of oxygen, known as superoxide radicals, roam the body leaving oxidative damage in their wake.

Oxidation is a daily assault that we all face. It's accelerated by smoking tobacco, having diabetes, or living in a polluted environment. Believed to play a critical role in the development of cardiovascular disease, cancer, cataracts, Parkinson's and Alzheimer's diseases, and amyotrophic lateral sclerosis (Lou Gehrig's disease), oxidative damage may be a central player in the aging process itself.

Enter antioxidants, compounds found in food that stop free-radical reactions and neutralize their destructive force. The antioxidants include vitamins C and E; carotenoids (certain pigments in vegetables and fruits that are precursors to vitamin A); flavonoids (found in delicacies from red wine to chocolate); indoles (plentiful in cruciferous vegetables like broccoli and cabbage); and the mineral selenium.

A number of studies have shown that individuals with high levels of antioxidants in their bloodstreams are protected from heart disease, cancer, and many of the diseases associated with oxidative damage. The question is, what's the best way to get antioxidants into your blood? The answer: Eat them in food! As with other nutrients, there's no good evidence that antioxidant supplements have the salubrious effect of eating them in your diet.

Vitamin C

One of the most familiar antioxidants is vitamin C. Very important to health and longevity, vitamin C can do far more than prevent scurvy—but not if you stop at the RDA of 60 milligrams a day designed to ward off that obsolete disease. Linus Pauling was the first to mount a major challenge to the RDA for vitamin C, and since he made a stir about the vitamin's potential in his book *Vitamin C and the Common Cold*, which was published in 1970, scientists have found that higher amounts of vitamin C in our diets may protect us from heart disease, stroke, cataracts, and certain cancers. Those who consume high levels of vitamin C may also be improving their memories and lung function.

Though Pauling popularized megadosing of vitamin C as a panacea against many ills, including the common cold (he took as much as 15,000 milligrams per day), research doesn't support this level of supplementation. For one thing, megadosing is a waste of money, since the body can only utilize 250 milligrams of vitamin C in a 24-hour cycle. Vitamin C can also increase the absorption of the oxidant mineral iron, of particular concern if you have hemochromatosis, a disorder of iron metabolism. Furthermore, there's a potential risk to taking megadoses of any given nutrient. And most important, there's no strong evidence that vitamin C from supplements provides the protection you get from eating it in food.

My AgeLess recommendation is to get 250 milligrams of vitamin C—more than four times the RDA—from food each day. Meeting this goal is easier than you might think. Just a glass of fresh orange juice, a serving of broccoli, and a cup of fresh strawberries will get you there. Vitamin C is widely available in foods, so you can get the AgeLess recommendation in your daily diet with just a little extra attention. (The table "Vitamin C" on page 244 shows some common dietary sources of C.) If you can't consume enough fruits and vegetables to get 250 milligrams, there is probably little harm in taking a daily 250-milligram vitamin C supplement. Note that this is four times the amount of vitamin C in the average multivitamin.

Colorful Carotenoids

The vivid colors of fruits and vegetables not only add visual appeal to produce bins but also can signal antioxidant-rich foods. Produce that's orange, dark yellow, dark green, or red is rich in carotenoids, colorful pigment compounds that act as powerful antioxidants. As I've mentioned, beta-carotene is the carotenoid that makes carrots orange. But don't look at skins and peels; it's the color of the flesh—the part you eat—that counts the most. A yellow-peeled banana is not high in carotenoids, but the orange flesh hidden behind the brown rind of a cantaloupe is. Here are some other foods with high carotenoid counts and their corresponding colors.

- ⑥ Orange: apricots, butternut squash, cantaloupe, carrots, mangoes, orange bell peppers, oranges, and pumpkins
- ⑥ Dark yellow: corn, papayas, peaches, sweet potatoes, and yellow bell peppers
- ⑥ Dark green: broccoli, collard greens, green bell peppers, kale, kiwifruit, romaine lettuce, spinach, and Swiss chard
- ⑥ Red: guava, pink grapefruit, red bell peppers, red grapes, tomatoes, and watermelon

The most common carotenoids are alpha- and beta-carotene, beta-cryptoxanthin, lycopene, lutein, and zeaxanthin.

Carotenoids can neutralize free radicals to help prevent cardiovascular disease and other diseases of aging. Overall, studies find that high levels of carotenoids in your diet can reduce your risk of heart disease by more than 35 percent, while people who eat lots of lycopene, the carotenoid in tomatoes, have a 50 to 60 percent decrease in their risk of heart disease. (More than 80 percent of Americans' lycopene consumption comes from tomato products, including ketchup, tomato juice, and pasta and pizza sauces. Cooking tomatoes releases their lycopene for better absorption, so a love of red sauces could lengthen your life.) In a 5-year study of 1,299 elderly Massachusetts residents, those participants who ate the most carotenoids in vegetables and fruits reduced their risk of death from cardiovascular disease by 45 percent.

Carotenoids may also help to prevent cancers of the lung, breast, prostate, cervix, skin, bladder, and digestive tract. In two large studies mentioned earlier, the Nurses' Health Study and the Health Professionals' Follow-Up Study, a diet rich in carotenoids lowered the risk of lung cancer by as much as 63 percent. High carotenoid levels have also been associated with the lowest risk of cervical cancer, and a lycopene-rich diet has been found to cut prostate cancer risk in half.

In the eye, retinal pigments derived from lutein and zeaxanthin transform light received by the retina into nerve signals to the brain. Eating lots of these carotenoids can protect against eye disease, including macular degeneration—the most common cause of blindness in older age—and cataracts, the main cause of reversible age-related vision loss.

The vitamin A derived from carotenoids in food appears to be far more beneficial and less hazardous than the retinol in vitamin A pills or multivitamins. Vitamin A supplements have also been associated with increased rates of hip fracture. In a recent study, women who took 10,000 IU of vitamin A per day—the amount found in some multivitamins—had an almost 50 percent higher risk of hip fractures over those who took the least vitamin A. Carotenoids in food can give you all the vitamin A you need without any risk of overdose—and though we don't know yet how many carotenoids are enough, there's no upper limit to how many you can safely eat in food.

Flavorful Flavonoids

Another family of healthy compounds found in fruits and vegetables are flavonoids. Your favorite flavonoids may include the resveratrol in red wine, catechins in your morning coffee or tea, quercetin in onions and apples, naringin in citrus fruits, isoflavones in soy, and—who knows?—maybe you've even enjoyed the lignans in flaxseed oil (it makes a great salad dressing). By far, though, the world's favorite flavonoids must be the catechins in chocolate.

Flavonoids are plant compounds with antioxidant effects. Chemi-

AgeLess Reward: The Three Cs

For the best protection against heart disease and cancer, choose the three Cs—cruciferous, citrus, and colorful produce. Here are the best ones.

- Cruciferous vegetables: bok choy, broccoli, Brussels sprouts, cabbage, cauliflower, and parsley
- Citrus fruits: grapefruit, oranges, and tangerines
- Orange and yellow vegetables and fruit: cantaloupe, carrots, mangoes, papaya, peaches, sweet potatoes, and winter squash

Measuring the Effects of Fruits and Vegetables

A study that compared people who ate 500 grams (18 ounces) of mixed fruits and vegetables a day with those who consumed just 100 grams (4 ounces) found significant differences in the amounts of nutrients circulating in their blood. On average, the 500-gram group's nutrient plasma levels were higher than the 100-gram group's by the following amounts:

Nutrient	% Increase
Alpha-carotene	121
Vitamin C	64
Lutein	46
Beta-carotene	45
Lycopene	22
Folate	15

The high-intake group also had lower levels of blood homocysteine, an amino acid that may contribute to heart disease and Alzheimer's disease (more on homocysteines later). The average homocysteine level of the people eating 500 grams of vegetables and fruits was 11 percent lower than that of the 100-gram group.

cally, they can inhibit the oxidation of LDL (low-density lipoprotein) cholesterol and reduce the tendency of blood to clot. Observational studies suggest that people who consume high levels of flavonoids have lower risks of cancers, heart disease, and stroke. Heed the beta-carotene story, however, before you rush out for flavonoid supplements. No evidence exists that these compounds are effective in the form of a pill. And why take a pill when a dark chocolate truffle tastes so much better?

Eat Chocolate, Live Longer?

It's no big surprise that the seed of the cocoa plant would have healthful properties, since many other plant seeds do, too (think beans and nuts). Dark chocolate is a rich source of catechins. These are the same flavonoids found in tea, but they're four times more concentrated in chocolate. And though chocolate is high in saturated fat, it appears that the stearic acid it contains does not have a negative impact on cholesterol; in fact, eating chocolate appears to improve cholesterol profiles.

A recent study put participants on two different diets, one including lots of dark chocolate and cocoa powder and the other low in all foods that contain flavonoids. The lucky chocolate group not only enjoyed the experience but also showed a boost in beneficial HDL cholesterol and a rise in the levels of antioxidants in their blood.

Another study took two groups of young men on a healthy diet and fed one a chocolate bar snack every day for a month, while the other group ate a chocolate-free snack. The groups switched snacks for another month, then the study team compared stats. When the men ate chocolate, they had higher good HDL cholesterol and lower bad triglyceride levels than when they snacked on nonchocolate foods.

Research on this sensual subject is still too limited to draw any firm conclusions, but many of us are keeping our fingers crossed for any reason to enjoy chocolate even more than before.

AgeLess Nutrition Is Easier Than It Seems

With all the different nutrients available in vegetables and fruits, it can be hard to remember their names, let alone the foods they appear in. If you find yourself in phytochemical overload (*phytochemical* is a general term for all the chemical compounds in plants), don't sweat the details. Instead, simply aim for the widest possible variety of plant foods in your diet and be sure to get your daily five-plus servings of fruits and veggies. Here are some fast and easy suggestions.

   ⊚ **Breakfast:** Start with a glass of orange juice, half a grapefruit, or a wedge of melon. Slice a banana or sprinkle berries over your cereal. Choose fresh fruit pancakes or waffles.

AgeLess Eating: Chocolate

For a high-quality chocolate indulgence, choose dark chocolate, which contains the highest concentrations of catechins (flavonoid compounds) and the least amount of fat.

The Antioxidant Kitchen

🌀 Cook tomatoes to maximize lycopene release. Make it pasta marinara tonight!—or enjoy some tomato soup, cooked tomato salsa, even ketchup (but be aware that this popular favorite contains a lot of sugar and salt).

🌀 Add a dash of olive oil to raise your carotenoid quotient. Carotenoids are fat-soluble, so you need a bit of fat in a meal in order to absorb them.

🌀 Sip a cup of green tea with honey for a tasty antioxidant cocktail.

🌀 Dip strawberries in dark chocolate for a double antioxidant dessert.

🌀 **Lunch:** Have a bowl of vegetable soup or a chopped salad. Most healthy brands of canned vegetable soup are packed with nutrients. Try fresh berries or melon for dessert.

🌀 **Dinner:** To put hot, steaming veggies on the table in minutes, pop them into a microwave-safe dish, cover with a lid or vented plastic wrap, add a splash of water, and cook until tender, for 1 to several minutes depending upon the type and amount. If steamed veggies aren't your style, grill, roast, or sauté them instead. Take advantage of convenient precleaned, packaged greens to enjoy a salad every day.

🌀 **Snacks:** Take a bag of apples to work. They're easy to eat out of hand without any peeling or mess. Keep a bag of baby carrots or some raw cauliflower on hand for snacks. Put out a fruit bowl and encourage the whole family to make it the first snack stop.

Fill Up on Fiber

If you need any more convincing about the importance of fruits and vegetables, let fiber make the argument. Absent in animal foods, fiber shows up only in plants—whole (unprocessed) grains, nuts, seeds, legumes, vegetables, and fruits. Fiber helps protect against heart disease, diabetes, digestive disorders, and perhaps cancer—and most Americans don't get enough.

The word *fiber* refers to several forms of complex carbohydrates that we can't digest. There are two main types, soluble and insoluble, and each plays a different role in preventing disease. Soluble fiber is the kind found in oat bran, legumes, nuts, and seeds. It is also found in pectin in apples and other fruits. Soluble fiber completely dissolves in the intestines where it acts to slow digestion and to help regulate blood sugar and cholesterol levels.

Insoluble fiber is what most folks think of as "roughage." Instead of dissolving in the system, insoluble fiber acts like a sponge to soak up water and speed the traffic of waste products, disposing of toxins before they can cause disease. Sources of insoluble fiber include whole grains, especially wheat bran, and *all fruits and vegetables*. These foods can relieve constipation and help to prevent diverticulosis, irritable bowel syndrome, and hemorrhoids.

In addition to maintaining your cardiovascular system, blood sugar balance, and digestive apparatus, fiber may also protect against peptic ulcer disease, hypertension, and cancers of the esophagus and pancreas. The preventive effect of fiber on colon cancer is still being debated— you've probably read the confusing headlines—but the fact remains that societies that eat high-fiber diets have lower cancer rates. We don't yet know whether this is a correlation or a cause-and-effect situation.

If you watch your weight, you'll know that fiber is a wonderful aid to appetite control, filling your stomach without adding a single calorie. Since it smooths out those blood sugar swings, soluble fiber can also keep you from running to the vending machine.

Fiber also tends to come in foods with other health-promoting properties, so the more fibrous your diet, the better. The rough stuff in whole grains may be particularly healthful. Most of us, however, are only halfway to making our daily fiber target. My AgeLess recommendation

Don't Do This

Plenty of folks look for their fruits and vegetables in all the wrong places. Do not count any of the following toward your daily quota.

- Fruit drinks, including many juice-bar offerings and smoothies. (These drinks are mostly sugar and water. Pure orange or grapefruit juice is fine.)
- French fries and potato chips. (They are soaked with transaturated or polysaturated fats and short on nutrients compared to many other vegetables.)
- Commercially prepared snack foods—fruit pies, bars, breakfast cereals, and pressed fruit rolls. (Where's the fruit?)
- Iceberg lettuce. (It has little nutrient value.)

Diverticulosis: The Disease You Don't Want but Are Likely to Get

How do you like the idea of small pockets bulging from the lining of your large intestine, filled with toxic waste? Half of all Americans have such pockets by age 60, and everybody has them by their 80th birthday. Eat enough fiber, and you can keep the pockets healthy and clean.

Diverticuli is the technical term for these intestinal bulges, and diverticulosis describes the condition of having them. When waste gets trapped inside diverticuli, the colon can become inflamed, causing diverticulitis, a disease characterized by cramping pain, possibly fever and nausea, and in the worst case rupture, which requires emergency surgery. Two hundred thousand Americans annually land in the hospital with this disease, which can clinically resemble appendicitis or ulcerative colitis. You're less likely to be among them if you get your daily dose of fiber.

Participants in the Harvard Nurses' Health Study who consumed the most insoluble fiber, particularly cellulose, cut their risk of diverticular disease by nearly half. Where to get cellulose? Fruits and veggies, of course.

(and that of the federal government) is to eat 25 grams of fiber a day, a little more than twice the national average of 11 grams a day. (See "Fiber" on page 247 for a listing of fiber-rich foods.)

Your diet should be your first source of fiber, but if you're falling short, fiber supplements, such as psyllium (Metamucil) and methylcellulose (Citrucel), are available to temporarily close the gap. But beware: Supplemental fiber lacks many of the healthful properties of whole foods. Furthermore, too much supplemental fiber can bind with critical nutrients and remove them from the body, which is not a concern with the natural fibers in food.

With any fiber supplement, water is critical! Skimp on your water intake, and you may find yourself constipated.

NEW NUTRITION RULE #3:
DON'T CUT BACK ON FATS— JUST CHOOSE THE RIGHT ONES

The fat-free revolution pioneered by Nathan Pritikin in the late '70s made fat "public enemy number one." Widely blamed for the nation's obesity epidemic and implicated in the high rates of heart disease and cancer, fat fell from grace with a resounding thud. But New Rule #3 gives food lovers something to cheer about: Not all fats are bad for you, and, in fact, some fats are beneficial. You do need to know the difference between them, however, and enjoy the right ones in moderation.

The fats you eat can affect your cholesterol ratio, which in turn determines your cardiovascular health and risk of heart attack, stroke, and peripheral artery disease. While cholesterol is necessary for life and naturally manufactured by the body, too much of the wrong kind can clog your arteries. LDL, a "bad" cholesterol, can become oxidized and start a chain reaction that results in the deposit of plaque onto arterial walls. Your goal is to lower your LDL cholesterol levels. HDL is "good" cholesterol that helps sweep LDL cholesterol out of the bloodstream. Generally, the higher your HDL cholesterol levels, the better.

Eating too many saturated fats (solid at room temperature) and transaturated fats, also called "trans fatty acids," (liquid fats hydrogenated to be solid at room temperature) can raise your LDL cholesterol level. The average American diet draws more than 30 percent of its calories from fat, and many of these are the saturated fats found in meat, butter, cream, lard, and cheese, or the related transaturated fats found in shortening, margarine, hydrogenated oils, commercially prepared baked goods, and deep-fried foods. Solid fat can stick to artery walls as surely as it spreads on bread, and this is true of Crisco, the marbling on steak, or the grease in an order of fries.

AGELESS TIP

Overcoming Fiber Phobia

If you tend to avoid fiber because of the noise it makes in your digestive system, try these tips.

- ⑥ Increase your fiber intake gradually and space high-fiber foods evenly throughout the day.
- ⑥ Drink plenty of water to rehydrate the fiber strands.
- ⑥ Try Beano, a digestive enzyme that helps process the complex sugars in fiber-rich foods such as beans, vegetables, and grains.

While it's been exciting to discover that cutting back on saturated fats can not only prevent but also reverse heart disease, the old rule—cut out fats—was a bitter pill for food lovers to swallow. This important finding has helped many people gain a new lease on life. Highly restrictive diets, however, like the one advocated by dietary pioneer Dr. Dean Ornish, who successfully treated heart disease with a super-lean regimen that limited fat to 10 percent of total calories, were hard to stick to, and dropping out was not the exception but the rule. Fortunately, the latest news is that you don't have to give up fats in order to save your heart. Several large studies, including the Nurses' Health Study and the Health Professionals' Follow-Up Study, found that the amount of fat consumption was not linked to heart disease risk, but the type of fat was. In these large studies, the more unsaturated fat in the participants' diets, the less their average risk of heart disease.

Monounsaturated fats protect your heart by boosting good HDL cholesterol and lowering bad LDL cholesterol. Make these your first choices; you'll find that the right fats are delicious additions to your healthy diet. Olive, canola, soybean, and flaxseed oils; almonds, peanuts, pecans, sesame seeds, sunflower seeds, and the oils made from all of them; and avocados are all good sources of monounsaturated fats. Then there are the omega-3 fatty acids, which we'll discuss in more detail on page 49. Common in fish and also found in walnuts and canola, flaxseed, and soybean oils, omega-3s seem to help keep your heart beating rhythmically. Finally, there are other health-promoting compounds in seed oils. Flaxseed oil contains alpha-linolenic acid, for instance, which helps to regulate blood pressure, and lignans, which are antioxidant compounds. Olive oil also offers the antioxidants vitamin E and polyphenols and appears to protect against colon cancer.

"I Can't Believe It's Not Butter!"

As you can see, plant fats are often good, animal fats always bad, and fish fats are nice if you can get them. Polyunsaturated plant fats such as corn and soybean oils are good in liquid form. Hydrogenating these liquid fats into solids, however, produces trans fats, which are even more deadly than saturated fat in your body, so margarine and vegetable shortening are definitely off the AgeLess list (except for a few new brands that are free of trans fats, like Smart Balance margarine).

Since AgeLess living is designed to optimize quality of life as well as its quantity, we can't neglect an important fact: Fat makes food taste better. It carries flavor molecules to aroma and taste receptors on the tongue and in the nose. (That's why some fat-free foods taste so flat.) Fat can help you feel satisfied with less food. You also need fat to absorb and transport fat-soluble vitamins and other life-extending nutrients and nourish healthy cells, skin, and hair. Eat and cook with mono- and polyunsaturated fats, and you do yourself and your food's flavor a favor. Here are some suggestions to get you started.

Ban butter from your sauté pan. Instead choose olive, canola, avocado, or peanut oil. Almond, sunflower, and other nut oils are alternatives. Try walnut, sesame, or hazelnut oil as a flavorful last-minute addition to your dish or as a base for salad dressings.

Use your head when you spread on bread. Whole grain toast, bread, bagels, and sandwiches can all meet the AgeLess nutrition requirements when you skip the butter, margarine, or full-fat cream cheese. Instead, choose peanut or other nut butters, fat-free or low-fat cream cheese, jelly or jam, tahini, hummus, trans-free margarine (such as Smart Balance), or mayonnaise. Dunk crusty multigrain bread in herbed olive oil for a Mediterranean-style treat. You won't miss the butter!

Bake better with oils. Many baked goods can be made with oil instead of butter, margarine, or shortening. You can also substitute Smart Balance when you want the texture of shortening.

Pick your protein. Avoid red meat and opt instead for skinless poultry, pork tenderloin, fish, or soy, legumes, and nuts.

Choose fat-free or low-fat dairy products. Substituting fat-free milk and low- or fat-free cheese, yogurt, and sour cream for their full-fat versions makes a big dip in your saturated fat intake while keeping your calcium intake high.

Remember that fat comes with a high calorie count. At nine calories per gram, it has more than double the four calories per gram found in carbohydrates and protein—so moderation is key. Match your caloric intake to your expenditure to prevent unwanted pounds.

Healthy Fats in Foods

My AgeLess recommendation is to eat and cook with monounsaturated fats. Here are some good sources of monounsaturated fats and omega-3 fatty acids.

Oils	Other Foods
Olive	Almonds (almond butter)
Canola	Peanuts (peanut butter)
Soybean	Pecans
Flaxseed	Sesame seeds (tahini)
Almond	Sunflower seeds
Hazelnut	Walnuts
Peanut	Avocados
Sesame	Fatty fish (salmon, sardines, mackerel, herring, tuna, rainbow trout)
Sunflower	
Walnut	
Avocado	

NEW NUTRITION RULE #4:
FOLLOW THE AGELESS NUTRITION PYRAMID

You're probably familiar with the Food Guide Pyramid created by the U.S. Department of Agriculture that pictures the elements of a healthy diet. New Rule #4 asks you to put that picture out of your head.

Created in 1992, the USDA Pyramid has come under fire since. Based on very little nutritional evidence at the time, it has been accused of representing special interests in the agriculture industry and encouraging the consumption of too many calories. With its heavy emphasis on eating refined starches and failure to point out important differences within food groups—for instance, between red meat and fish or saturated and monounsaturated fats—the USDA Pyramid was flawed even by old standards. It doesn't begin to represent what we know now. Enter the AgeLess Nutrition Pyramid: I've created a new hierarchy based on foods that will nourish your healthspan.

The AgeLess Nutrition Pyramid shows how to apply the New Nutrition Rules to your daily meal plan. The AgeLess diet is similar to the traditional Mediterranean diet, which, compared to the average Amer-

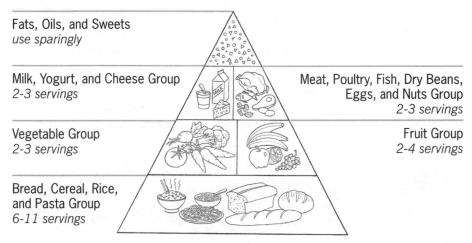

Fats, Oils, and Sweets
use sparingly

Milk, Yogurt, and Cheese Group
2-3 servings

Meat, Poultry, Fish, Dry Beans,
Eggs, and Nuts Group
2-3 servings

Vegetable Group
2-3 servings

Fruit Group
2-4 servings

Bread, Cereal, Rice,
and Pasta Group
6-11 servings

USDA Food Guide Pyramid

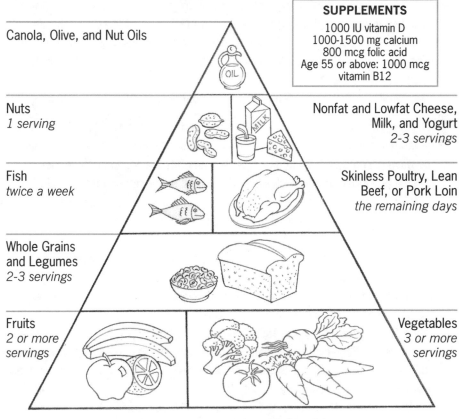

Canola, Olive, and Nut Oils

SUPPLEMENTS

1000 IU vitamin D
1000-1500 mg calcium
800 mcg folic acid
Age 55 or above: 1000 mcg
vitamin B12

Nuts
1 serving

Nonfat and Lowfat Cheese,
Milk, and Yogurt
2-3 servings

Fish
twice a week

Skinless Poultry, Lean
Beef, or Pork Loin
the remaining days

Whole Grains
and Legumes
2-3 servings

Fruits
*2 or more
servings*

Vegetables
*3 or more
servings*

AgeLess Nutrition Pyramid

ican diet, features more green and root vegetables, more whole grain bread, more fish, less red meat, fruit at least once a day, lots of olive oil for cooking, and wine in moderation. Some of the first hints we had of the power of diet to optimize longevity were statistics coming out of Mediterranean countries. Though residents of these countries were hardly paragons of good health—they smoked more and exercised less than Americans, for example—they had lower rates of

DR. WALTER WILLETT'S

Top 10 Tips for Happy, Healthy Eating

Walter Willett, M.D., knows a lot about eating well. As a professor of epidemiology and nutrition and chairman of the department of nutrition at Harvard School of Public Health, he was one of the first to point out and correct problems with the USDA's Food Guide Pyramid and encourage Americans to use their daily diets as a route to better health. He's been a leader in large epidemiological studies of diet and health, including the Nurses' Health Study and the Health Professionals' Follow-Up Study, which you've read about throughout this chapter.

Here are Dr. Willett's top 10 tips for eating your way to a longer healthspan.

1. **Choose good fats.** Replace saturated and trans fats (from partially hydrogenated vegetable oils) with healthy unsaturated fats. Butter and red meat are the main sources of saturated fats, while trans fats are found in some margarines and most commercial baked goods and fast food. Almost all liquid vegetable oils can help reduce high blood cholesterol levels and heart disease risk. Of course, too much of a good thing can lead to weight gain, so don't overdo good fats.

2. **Include omega-3 fatty acids each day.** Fish is an excellent source of these polyunsaturated fats, which can reduce the likelihood of fatal rhythm disturbances of the heart. Canola and soybean oils, flaxseed, flaxseed oil, and walnuts are also good sources of omega-3 fatty acids.

3. **Minimize refined starches.** These include white bread, white rice, white pasta, and potatoes. Replacing these refined starches with their whole grain counterparts adds important micronutrients and fiber, aids bowel function, reduces risk of heart disease, and may help in weight control.

4. **Minimize sugar.** Many beverages and "low-fat" foods contain large amounts of

heart disease and cancer. The key longevity factor appeared to be diet.

Since the scientific community first took note of the Mediterranean diet, epidemiological studies and controlled interventions alike have proven its health benefits. The results of this work are encapsulated in the New Rules to create a science-based plan for living la dolce vita.

Like the USDA pyramid, the AgeLess Nutrition Pyramid reads from the bottom up to show the correct proportions of the different food

---

sugar, which provide empty calories. Even natural fruit juices are full of sugar and are best limited to one small glass per day.

5. **Select healthy protein sources.** Nuts, beans, and soy products can meet your protein needs if you want to be a vegetarian, but fish and chicken add variety to your meals and can be just as healthy. If you like red meat, limit it to once or twice per week.

6. **Enjoy an abundance of vegetables and fruits.** The health benefits are many, and they add variety and interest to any diet.

7. **Get enough folic acid.** You'll find folate, the natural form of folic acid, in many fruits and vegetables, but taking a folic acid supplement is a good way to be sure that your intake is adequate.

8. **Don't fall short on vitamin D.** If you live in the southern United States and spend time in the sunshine regularly, vitamin D deficiency should be no problem. For those of us in the north, however, where sunshine is weak during the winter or for people who live in an indoor, air-conditioned world, supplemental vitamin D makes sense.

9. **Consider your alcohol consumption carefully.** Moderate alcohol consumption (two or fewer drinks per day) decreases risks of heart disease and probably diabetes, but high intake has many known adverse effects. Some people should not drink at all if there is reason to suspect a risk for alcoholism.

10. **Be an adventuresome eater.** The last decades of research have shown that healthy diets need not be dull or boring. Dozens of cultures around the world have learned to piece together the elements described above in thousands of ways that are attractive and tasty as well as healthy, and creative cooks are continually finding new ways to do this.

For Dr. Willett's comprehensive advice about eating for health and vitality, including recipes, menus, and tips, see his book *Eat, Drink, and Be Healthy: The Harvard Medical School Guide to Healthy Eating (Simon & Schuster)*.

groups. Vegetables and fruits come first, followed by whole grains and legumes, fish, lean poultry, nuts, fat-free and low-fat dairy products, and unsaturated fats. These are not your grandmother's food groups!—unless, of course, your grandmother came from one of the Mediterranean countries!

Get Whole Grains

Although "amber waves of grain" is a cherished American image, to many modern Americans it's an outdated one. Nowadays, food manufacturers strip most whole grains down to a nutrient-depleted white powder before we eat them. The practice is not good for our health. The bran removed when whole grains are refined is rich in folate, vitamin E and other antioxidants, and fiber. Most nutritionists recommend that we eat three servings each day, for good reason. In one study, women who ate the most whole grains had a 30 percent lower risk of heart disease.

Unfortunately, with our taste for highly refined starches, it's hard to find an American who gets those three daily servings. In fact, the national average is just one serving every 2 days! In his book, *Eat, Drink, and Be Healthy,* Harvard nutrition expert Walter Willett, M.D., offers three reasons for the lack of whole grains in our diets: We're not familiar with most whole grains, it's harder to find them in grocery stores, and they take longer to cook. Yet it's worth making the effort. Most people would get their recommended servings simply by substituting whole grains for the refined grains they already eat. The extra bonus is that you eliminate a lot of empty calories this way.

Love Your Legumes

Another longevity-boosting food is the legume—technically, a plant seed that comes in a pod. You may know them as beans. Indeed, included in the legume family are beans, lentils, peanuts, and peas. Legumes are excellent sources of soluble fiber, folate, and plant protein, and they are every bit as heart-healthy as that suggests.

Eating legumes can lower your LDL cholesterol level, since their soluble fiber slows down the absorption of cholesterol. As mentioned earlier, soluble fiber also improves blood sugar control, making it a boon for people with diabetes, as it has been found to improve blood sugar control. The folate in beans can help lower homocysteine levels

Whole Grain Substitutes for Refined Grains

My AgeLess recommendation is to substitute whole grains for refined grains and get at least 2 to 3 total servings of whole grains and/or legumes per day.

Substitute Whole Grains . . .	For Refined Grains . . .
Breads	
Whole wheat and other whole grain breads	White bread
	White bread dyed brown
Breakfast	
Whole grain breakfast cereal (Cheerios, cornflakes, bran, and others)	Refined grain breakfast cereal
Cooked oatmeal	Pancakes
Bran muffins	Waffles
	English muffins
	Blueberry muffins
	Bagels
Pasta, side dishes, casseroles	
Brown rice	White rice
Bulgar	Regular pasta and noodles
Quinoa	
Whole wheat pasta	
Snacks	
Popcorn	Cake
Baked corn chips	Cookies
Baking	
Whole wheat flour	White flour
Wheat germ	
Oatmeal	
Cornmeal	
Wheat or oat bran	

Legumes for Longevity

My AgeLess recommendation is to eat at least 2 to 3 servings of legumes and/or whole grains such as these a day.

- ⑥ Beans (black, white, navy, pinto, kidney, fava, and others)
- ⑥ Lentils
- ⑥ Lima beans
- ⑥ Peanuts
- ⑥ Peas (green, black-eyed, split, and others)

(more on this coming up), while getting protein from beans instead of meat is a good way to reduce your intake of saturated fat.

No wonder people who eat a lot of legumes have a lower risk of heart disease. A 19-year follow-up of the National Health and Nutrition Examination Survey (NHANES) tracked nearly 10,000 men and women and found that the more legumes they ate, the less likely they were to develop heart disease. Those who helped themselves to a serving of beans or other legumes four or more times per week lowered their heart disease risk by 22 percent.

Because legumes and whole grains are both high-fiber carbohydrate sources, I use them interchangeably in my AgeLess recommendation of 2 to 3 servings per day. Here are a few ideas for upping your bean count. Try the following:

- ⑥ Bean chili
- ⑥ Hummus
- ⑥ Minestrone
- ⑥ Many Mexican dishes (but watch the lard and cheese)
- ⑥ Split pea soup
- ⑥ Baked beans
- ⑥ Soy burgers
- ⑥ Bean salads

Go Nuts!

Nuts are the new kids on the foods for longevity block. Like their cousins the legumes, these seeds of trees are equipped with the nutrition to start new life. Even the nuts' fat turns out to be a key nutritional asset. The fat in nuts is almost all unsaturated and much of it is monounsaturated, the type that can improve your cholesterol profile. Many nuts, especially walnuts, also contain heart-healthy omega-3 fatty acids. Nuts' other nutritional advantages include antioxidants—flavonoids, vitamin E, the mineral selenium, and ellagic acid—lots of fiber (2.5 grams in a single ounce), and plant protein.

Epidemiological studies show that people who eat the most nuts have a 20 to 50 percent lower risk of heart disease than the rest. For instance, among the 85,000 participants in the Harvard Nurses' Health Study, those who ate five or more weekly servings of nuts had a third lower risk of heart disease over the study's 14-year period than the nurses who said "no" to nuts. Another study by the Harvard School of Public Health estimated that substituting the fat in 1 ounce of nuts for the equivalent amount of saturated fat can lower the risk of coronary heart disease by 45 percent. Eating nuts may even improve the health of people who already follow a Mediterranean-style diet. In a small study in Spain of 50 people with high cholesterol, researchers found that substituting walnuts for 35 percent of their calories from monounsaturated fat lowered total and LDL cholesterol levels by an average of 4 to 6 percent.

My AgeLess recommendation is to eat five 1-ounce servings of nuts per week. Your best bets for AgeLess eating in the nut family include:

- Walnuts
- Cashews
- Pecans
- Pistachios
- Almonds
- Peanuts (actually a legume)

Ultimate New Rules: Nutty Chocolate Snack

When walnuts meet dark chocolate, tastebuds rejoice! And in moderation, this combination can improve your longevity quotient with antioxidants, fiber, and omega-3 fatty acids. To make your own chocolate-covered walnuts, toast walnut halves in a 350°F oven until fragrant, dip in melted dark chocolate. Cool on waxed paper until the chocolate rehardens. Enjoy!

Say "No" to Coconuts

Though its name says "nut," coconut is actually the fruit of the palm tree. It has none of the healthful benefits of either fruit or nuts. In fact, coconut flesh is packed with saturated fat—4 grams in a mere 2 tablespoons of flakes.

Say "Yes" to Seafood

When choosing a protein, many Americans think first of red meat—but it should be clear by now that this isn't the best choice for optimal longevity. Don't worry—I'm not going to make you become a vegetarian, though if you are one that's fine. I simply ask that you shift your protein choices toward fish, seafood, skinless poultry, and vegetable protein—and if you're a die-hard red meat lover, toward pork tenderloin and specially bred lean beef.

First on the list of reasons to limit red meat consumption is the saturated fat it contains, with its attendant contribution to high LDL cholesterol levels and increased risk of heart disease. In addition to hardening your arteries, a diet containing lots of red meat has been linked with increased risk of colon, breast, pancreatic, and prostate cancers. The factors here may include not only saturated fat but also the charred compounds formed when fatty meats are cooked over high heat. Called heterocyclic amines, these chemicals, which form the toasty crust on your short ribs, are believed to be carcinogenic. You can minimize heterocyclic amine formation by baking, boiling, poaching, or braising meats instead of broiling, grilling, or sautéing them over high heat. There's no guarantee, however, that such cooking methods weaken the red meat–cancer connection, nor do they make the saturated fat in meat less menacing to your heart.

So make your next steak a salmon steak instead. Since the 1970's, when studies found that the fish-eating Inuit people of Greenland had an unusually low rate of heart disease, we've collected lots of data showing the health benefits of regular fish consumption. In fact, several studies show that people who eat at least one serving of fish each week have half the risk of dying from a heart attack.

These benefits seem attributable to the fact that fish have next to no saturated fat. Even shellfish, which are high in cholesterol, score close to zero on saturated fat, so they don't pose a problem to the cholesterol level in your blood, which responds more to the amount of saturated fat—rather than cholesterol—you eat.

The type of fat that fish *do* have actually contributes to your longevity and health. Long-chain polyunsaturated fatty acids are the fats found in fish. Of particular interest are the omega-3 fatty acids, including docosahexaenoic acid (DHA) and eicosapentaenoic acid (EPA). I'll just call these omega-3s.

Omega-3 fatty acids can lower triglycerides, prevent blood clots, and (this is what sets them apart) act as a check on electrical misfires in your heartbeat to prevent heart attacks. As one measure of this effect, researchers took a sample of participants from the Physicians' Health Study and found that the men with the highest levels of omega-3 fatty acids in their blood at the beginning of the study had a 70 percent lower risk of sudden cardiac death over the next 10 years. Since our bodies don't make omega-3s, we need an outside source: Eating them in fish is a good plan. Furthermore, it doesn't take much fish to do the trick. It seems that just one or two weekly servings are enough; eating more doesn't further lower your heart attack risk. In fact, you probably don't want to eat too much fish overall, since some species, such as shark, swordfish, and striped bass, can be contaminated with mercury. Pregnant women should have no more than two servings of fish per week to minimize potential fetal exposure to mercury.

For omega-3 protection, choose fatty fish from cold, deep waters.

Fish Rich in Omega-3s

My AgeLess recommendation is to eat two servings of fatty fish per week.

First Choice Fish (high in omega-3s)	Omega-3 Content (grams in a 3½-ounce serving)
Salmon	2.3
Sardines	2.2
Mackerel	2.0
Herring	2.0
Tuna	1.6
Rainbow trout	1.2

These include salmon, albacore and bluefin tuna, sablefish, Atlantic mackerel, herring, sardines, bluefish, sturgeon, and lake trout. Shellfish and white-fleshed fish, on the other hand, have hardly any omega-3s.

Longevity Libations

Food's natural partner is drink. With what should you wash down an AgeLess meal?

AgeLess people don't sip much on soft drinks, which score a zero for your longevity quotient for having too much sugar and no nutritional value. Fat-free milk is a great choice as a source of calcium (coming up) and protein. Coffee and tea offer flavonoids and are fine in moderation. A daily toast with wine, beer, or alcohol may also give a

The Dean's Dozen:
12 Top Foods for Longevity

Food	AgeLess Advantages
Olive oil	Monounsaturated fats
Nuts	Can lower risk of heart disease; raise HDL and lower LDL cholesterol levels; provide vitamin E, fiber, and plant protein
Salmon	Omega-3-fatty acids and vitamin D
Fat-free yogurt	Calcium and vitamin D with little lactose
All-Bran cereal	Cereal fiber
Legumes (pick one: beans, lentils, split peas)	Folate, fiber, plant protein
Cruciferous vegetables (pick one: broccoli, cauliflower, cabbage)	Carotenoids, flavonoids, indoles, vitamin C, fiber
Spinach	Lutein, zeaxanthin, folate, fiber
Cooked tomatoes	Lycopene, fiber, vitamin C
Oranges	Vitamin C, fiber, folate
Berries (pick one: blueberries, strawberries, raspberries)	Vitamin C, fiber, antioxidants
Dark chocolate (in moderation)	Flavonoids, great taste!

Fast Food Can Dehydrate You

Fast food can be hard on your health in many ways. Scientists have now discovered that a typical fast-food meal of a burger and soft drink can cause dehydration, with consequences from cramps and impaired performance to worse.

The dehydrators in America's favorite meal are the protein in the burger and the caffeine and carbonation in the soft drink. Digesting protein requires a good deal of water, which is then flushed out of the body to eliminate waste by-products. (This accounts for the illusory initial weight loss you can get from a high-protein diet.) Caffeine compounds the water loss, acting as a diuretic to speed the flow of urine. Meanwhile, the carbonation in soft drinks can cause bloating, which makes you feel full and discourages you from drinking water to replace what you lost.

It was former tennis star Jimmy Connors's debilitating cramps on the court that got doctors started on this line of investigation. Connors was quite a cola drinker, and his example proves the rule that water is the best hydrator for performance and health.

boost to your healthspan if you already imbibe. But the very best longevity "potion" comes from the original fountain of youth: pure, clear water.

The world's greatest hydrator, water costs little and has no calories or side effects. Our bodies are composed mainly of water—you're carrying around about 10 gallons inside your body right now—and you need plenty of it to keep things running smoothly. Without fluids, you'd soon be dead, generally within a few days. Water's main jobs are to regulate your body's internal temperature and flush toxins out of the system. Hardworking H_2O also helps to reduce your risk of bladder and colon cancers. The waste products in urine and stool contain carcinogens, and the longer they stay in the body, the more likely they are to do harm. Drinking plenty of fluids speeds waste out of the body, minimizing your exposure.

Drinking plenty of water also prevents kidney stones. A kidney stone is a precipitate of minerals that forms in the kidney and then may pass through the ureter, bladder, and urethra on its way out of the body, an agonizing journey that ranks right up there with the pain of childbirth. Drinking enough water can wash these minerals away before they form a stone as well as flush smaller stones out of your body. Water also expands fiber in your digestive system so it can do its job, plumps up your skin, and keeps you feeling full.

While all beverages contain water, pure H_2O is best for hydration. As for your beloved latte or iced tea, the caffeine in these drinks acts as a diuretic, so drinking coffee, tea, or caffeinated soft drinks can actually dehydrate rather than rehydrate you.

Monitoring your fluid intake becomes even more important with age. You've heard the news stories about seniors succumbing to heatstroke during the dog days of summer. This susceptibility develops as we grow older, when the part of the brain that regulates thirst becomes less sensitive and starts failing to signal us to drink. Meanwhile, kidney function also becomes less precise, and your kidneys eliminate more water than they should. The combination of water loss and lower intake can lead to dehydration, which, when mild, impairs cognitive and physical function and, at higher levels, can be deadly. No matter what your age, get in the habit of drinking as much water as you can and keep with it.

How much H_2O is enough? Though many books and articles promote drinking eight glasses of water a day, there is little scientific evidence to support this recommendation. A good rule of thumb is that if you feel thirsty, you're already fluid-deficient. One of the simplest life-extending habits you can establish is learning to live without thirst by drinking water throughout the day and upping the amount when you exercise and in warm weather.

AGELESS MYTH BUSTER

Bottled Water

MYTH

Bottled water is better than tap water.

FACT

You can choose designer water for its taste or the trendy bottle it comes in, but most bottled waters offer no more health benefits than what comes out of your faucet. Water, however, that comes from protected underground sources and/or has been filtered may contain fewer contaminants than tap water, so if you're going to pay for fancy H_2O, look for this information on the label.

Alcohol: A Toast to Longevity?

The more you lift your water glass, the better—but what about stronger stuff? People have toasted life with alcohol for the past 10,000 years or more, and it looks as if light drinking may offer longevity benefits for some people. Heavy drinking, though, definitely decreases your chances of aging well, and binge drinking is even worse. An AgeLess relationship with alcohol relies upon moderation and consistency.

Many studies have found an inverse relationship between moderate drinking, defined as one to two drinks per day, and risk of coronary artery disease and stroke. One study that followed 490,000 men and women, ages 30 to 104(!), for 9 years found a 30 to 40 percent reduction in heart disease mortality among those of either sex who had at least one drink a day over those who were teetotalers. When it comes to alcohol, less is clearly more, though. In fact, this study found that the lowest rate of mortality from all causes was among people who reported having about one drink a day. Another study of stroke identified the greatest risk reduction—25 percent—among men who had just two to four drinks a week.

Alcohol's happy effect on the heart stems from the biochemical changes it causes. The next time you lift a glass, you can toast to the boost you're about to give to your good HDL cholesterol levels. You can also celebrate the fact that your blood will soon be less likely to clot, and that you're giving your body a break from stress. Make all three toasts in the space of one drink and stop there.

Any type of alcohol can have these effects, so it doesn't matter whether your drink of choice is a single-malt scotch, buttery Chardonnay, or beer in a can. The discovery of antioxidant flavonoid compounds in red wine has led to some speculation that this particular tipple offers additional health benefits, but before you start stocking your wine cellar, be advised that we don't yet have enough strong data to support this.

All that said, there are some important caveats about alcohol and aging well. Drinking more than one drink a day appears to increase the risk of breast cancer, so women should be especially careful about not exceeding that amount. In both men and women, heavy alcohol consumption is associated with increased risk for cancers of the mouth, esophagus, pharynx, larynx, and liver; accidents; and, if abused, with cirrhosis, brain cell death, and a host of other medical, personal, and social problems.

If you already drink alcohol, my AgeLess recommendation is to stick to the one-drink-a-day limit. Drinking more than that will cause you to age more.

TAKE ONLY THE SUPPLEMENTS YOU NEED

Notwithstanding my New Rule to toss your multivitamin and most supplements, there are three important nutrients that are just too hard to get from food in adequate amounts, no matter how carefully we plan our diets. They are calcium, vitamin D, and folic acid. (Vitamin B_{12} joins the AgeLess supplement list when you hit age 55.)

Calcium: You Never Outgrow Your Need for It

Between the ages of 5 and 10, my youngest son broke bones twice, and in neither case did he even miss a day of school. My 91-year-old mother, on the other hand, has broken her hip four times and is now in a nursing home, unable to walk or care for herself without help. George Burns was one of the liveliest nonagenarians around, but he died within a year of breaking his hip. The Pope himself had to cut back on his vigorous schedule after suffering a hip fracture. Strong bones are absolutely essential to successful aging, and calcium is the mineral that maintains them.

Calcium also protects against heart disease, stroke, colon cancer, and perhaps other diseases of aging. This mighty mineral is a New Rules essential, and you need to concentrate on getting your daily dose.

Bone Basics

The bones in your body are continuously remodeling themselves. Inside your skeleton are cells called osteoblasts that create new bone, and cells that remove bone, called osteoclasts. During the first part of your life the osteoblasts take the lead, building bone faster than the osteoclasts can take it away. After about age 30, though, the osteoclasts gain the upper hand and start draining density from your bones in a slow decline that lasts for the rest of your life. For women, this bone loss accelerates after menopause. Both sexes can slow the loss with weight bearing exercise.

Declining bone density results in weak, brittle bones, classified as osteoporosis when your bone mass is two standard deviations below the peak for your gender. Brittle bones break easily, and by age 65, your chances of sustaining a hip fracture are significantly increased. A hip fracture can rob you of your mobility and start you down the road to disability and death. Of the 300,000 Americans a year who suffer hip fractures, more than 20 percent don't survive a year; another 25 percent never walk again unassisted.

No matter what your age is now, you must start preventing serious bone breaks *today*. Calcium is key.

Calcium is not only the primary component of bones, but our bodies also require it for many other biological functions. When you don't take in enough dietary calcium to support all these operations, your body takes it from your bones. This tactic may avert an immediate biochemical crisis, but it's disastrous to long-term bone health. Once the osteoclasts start working faster than the osteoblasts, your bones never get that borrowed calcium back. That's why you must get enough calcium to meet your body's needs every single day.

Once thought to be chiefly important to building bones, calcium is now believed to provide an array of other health benefits. Evidence suggests that calcium may play key roles in lowering blood pressure, preventing heart disease and stroke, and reducing risk of colon cancer.

Got Calcium?

Because calcium has so much work to do, we need a lot of it, and most American adults fall short of the recommended dietary allowance (1,000 to 1,500 milligrams, depending on gender and age).

Recommended Total Daily Intake of Calcium

These are the dietary reference intakes for calcium from the federal government. Men and women alike are advised to increase calcium intake with age.

Age	Women	Men
25–50	1,000 mg	1,000 mg
50–65	1,500 mg	1,000 mg
Over 65	1,500 mg	1,500 mg

Source: Dietary Reference Intakes, National Academy of Sciences, Washington, D.C.

On average, we obtain only 50 to 70 percent of this much calcium through food. It takes five glasses of milk a day to make a calcium target of 1,500 milligrams, and most of us choose something else to drink instead, so this shortfall isn't too surprising. Lots of great foods contain calcium, however. Dairy products—milk, yogurt, cheese—rank number one, followed (after a steep drop-off) by foods such as oatmeal, almonds, soy, and leafy greens. For a complete list, see "Calcium" on page 248.

The best way to get enough calcium is to eat plenty of calcium-rich foods. Choose low-fat or fat-free dairy products, since whole milk contains saturated fat. If you're lactose intolerant, take the enzyme supplement Lactaid when you eat dairy products, or look for Lactaid milk. You may be able to tolerate yogurt or cheese (semisoft to hard), since they are made using a fermentation process that eats up most of the lactose sugars.

Vegans who avoid dairy can get calcium from oatmeal, legumes (especially soybeans and tofu), leafy greens, or nuts. Unfortunately, the bioavailability of calcium from plant foods is low. Spinach, for instance, is full of calcium but contains a compound that inhibits its digestion, as does wheat bran. These are great foods in other regards, so eat them—but don't include them in your calcium calculations.

My AgeLess recommendation is to meet your calcium requirement with food and supplements. By all means, eat plenty of calcium-rich foods, but most of you will need to take a supplement in order to get 1,000 to 1,500 milligrams daily. There aren't many downsides to taking extra calcium, and the upside can be significant, so I recommend calcium supplementation with some important caveats.

First, consult with your doctor before taking calcium supplements if you take prescription drugs or have kidney stones. Like many supplements, calcium can interfere with other medications, particularly

Ultimate AgeLess Refresher: The Two Cs

Try calcium-enriched orange juice for a refresher rich in two key nutrients: calcium and vitamin C.

tetracycline, so be sure to check on the effect of calcium on all your prescription drugs. Certain types of kidney stones can be made worse with calcium supplements, though recent evidence indicates that there's no problem if you have the most common kind. Those free of this painful condition will be glad to know that consuming calcium is one of the best ways to help prevent kidney stones in the first place.

Next, because calcium is available in a variety of forms, choose the type of calcium to take. I recommend calcium citrate. It's the most easily absorbed form of supplemental calcium, and it doesn't cause constipation, as calcium carbonate can. Unlike some other forms, calcium citrate doesn't reduce the absorption of iron.

Finally, look for the amount of *elemental calcium* in your supplement, which is not necessarily the same as the number on the front of the bottle. This is the figure that counts in fulfilling your AgeLess recommendation. You can absorb only 500 milligrams of calcium at a time, so space out your supplements and calcium-rich foods through the day. And don't forget to get enough vitamin D, which is critical to calcium absorption. (More on this coming up.)

You should take the maximum calcium recommendation (1,500 mg) if you regularly consume large quantities of caffeine, sodium, or protein. Each of these speeds calcium loss.

Vitamin D: Calcium's Best Buddy

Vitamin D transports calcium from the intestine into your bloodstream. Without it, you would absorb a mere 10 percent of the calcium you ingest, which is why we now fortify milk with D. Misnamed long ago "vitamin," D is actually a hormone. Like other hormones, your body can manufacture D, but only with a little help from the sun.

Do you remember photosynthesis, the process that allows plants to convert sunlight to energy? The way humans create vitamin D from the rays of the sun is strikingly alike, though in this case it's called photolysis. Your skin contains a precursor to vitamin D, a chemical called 7-dehydrocholesterol. When the ultraviolet-B photons in sunlight penetrate the skin, they set off a series of chemical reactions that ends with the formation of the active form of vitamin D. It's an amazing phenomenon; you're nourished by the light!

D Is Our Number One Deficiency

Vitamin D is the most common vitamin deficiency in the United States. Present and future, this deficiency is a threat to your healthspan. In addition to keeping bones strong, vitamin D may play a role in preventing cancers of the breast, prostate, and colon. Low levels of D have been associated with risk for these diseases.

Why such a widespread shortfall? Indoor work deprives us of regular exposure to the sun, and vitamin D is virtually nonexistent in food. The only significant dietary source of vitamin D isn't even natural—it's milk fortified with synthetic D. It was a great idea when the dairy industry decided to team up vitamin D with the calcium in milk, but you'd still have to drink eight glasses of milk a day to make the AgeLess recommendation for vitamin D. Cod-liver oil (ick!) and lots of oily fish are your only other options.

Vitamin D deficiency is even more widespread among older adults, as the body's ability to synthesize sunlight declines. At age 21, spending just 3 to 5 minutes outside three times a week with your face, arms, and hands exposed can deliver your full D dose—and at that point in life you're probably catching plenty of rays. By age 65, however, depletion of the skin chemical that is converted to vitamin D means that you may need a total of 45 minutes outside on the week's sunniest days to synthesize adequate amounts of vitamin D.

No matter what your age, no one who lives as far north as New York, Chicago, or Seattle can get adequate D during winter. Other factors in your personal photolysis equation include your skin pigmenta-

Location Matters: D-Deficient Sun Zones

Does the sun shine enough where you live to synthesize the vitamin D you need? Not during the winter if you're above 40 degrees latitude north—which includes a third of the United States, all of Canada, and most of Europe—or below 40 degrees south. Some cities where the winter sun is too weak to scare up any D at all include Barcelona, Beijing, Berlin, Boston, Chicago, London, Montreal, Moscow, New York, Paris, Portland, Seattle, Stockholm, Rome, and Toronto. We who live in Los Angeles may take some ribbing on other fronts, but we're doing great on our vitamin D!

Weekly Sun Exposure
Recommendation for Vitamin D

My AgeLess recommendation is to get 1,000 IU of vitamin D a day from supplements and/or sun exposure. Do not exceed 1,000 IU a day from supplements.

Use these guidelines for getting your vitamin D from the sun. Keep in mind that the sun isn't strong enough to trigger vitamin D production during the winter at high latitudes.

Age	Weekly Sun Exposure (without sunscreen, with face and arms exposed)*
Under 65	3–5 minutes, 2–3 times a week
65 and above	5–15 minutes, 2–3 times a week

* Individuals at high risk for skin cancer should have no sun exposure without sunscreen.

tion, use of sunscreen, the season, the time of day, and the amount of ozone in the atmosphere. With all these variables, it's easy to wind up deficient in D.

The dietary reference intakes (DRIs) for vitamin D start at 200 IU and range up to 600 IU in older ages. Prominent researchers on vitamin D, however, recommend a daily intake of 1,000 IU to prevent deficiency and provide vitamin D's important health benefits. Few people reach this goal through sun exposure and fortified foods and need to take D in supplemental form. Since toxicity doesn't set in until doses well over 2,400 IU, I've set the AgeLess recommendation for vitamin D at 1,000 IU for all ages unless you're getting the sun exposure outlined in "Weekly Sun Exposure Recommendation for Vitamin D" above. Most multivitamins provide 400 IU, which might work if you're young

AGELESS TIP
Fishing for Vitamin D

Fish are one of the few good food sources of vitamin D. Five ounces of salmon provides 400 IU of D, which is almost half of the AgeLess recommendation.

and on the sunny side of the street but falls short for many folks, especially seniors.

As a fat-soluble substance, vitamin D can build up in fatty tissues and accumulate to toxic levels. While the body has natural protective mechanisms that prevent you from making too much vitamin D from sunlight, supplements aren't discriminating, and toxic levels could build up in your body. Therefore, it's important not to oversupplement with vitamin D. Cap your dose at my recommendation of 1,000 milligrams per day.

Catching Rays: Be Smart About It

People are often surprised when I tell them to get more sun. But when you worship the sun wisely, you age better on a few different fronts. Make light of this powerful force, though, and your healthspan will suffer.

Sun exposure ages your skin, and the consequence can be cancer at worst and wrinkles, discoloration, and age spots in less serious scenarios. The sun can also age your eyes. People who spend a lot of time in the sun without proper sunglasses are more likely to develop cataracts. On the other hand, besides generating vitamin D, sunlight can increase your healthspan by improving sleep and lifting mood. How can you reconcile my AgeLess recommendation with what your dermatologist and ophthalmologist may tell you?

Buyer Beware

One reason to exercise caution when taking dietary supplements is that many of them are not what they claim to be. The FDA has little power to regulate supplements, and, as a result, everything from the strength of a product to its ingredients and impurities may be misrepresented on labels and in ads.

In one sad case published in *The New England Journal of Medicine*, a man taking a vitamin D supplement labeled as 6,000 IU (way too high to begin with!) wound up in the hospital with vitamin D toxicity. Lab analysis of his supplements indicated that they may have contained more than 2 million IU of vitamin D.

AGELESS TIP

Vitamin D Blockers

Warning: It's difficult to catch photolysis-inducing rays through a window or layer of sunscreen. Glass and sunscreen both block UVB rays, so sunlight through a closed window or on your lotion-covered skin won't contribute much toward your vitamin D quota.

The following four principles will help keep your skin and eyes safe and your vitamin D levels healthy.

Let your skin show. The chemical reaction you seek can't happen unless sunlight hits the skin on your face, arms, and hands. Even in the sun-drenched country of Lebanon, vitamin D deficiency has been found among Islamic women who follow the dress code requiring their legs, arms, and head to be covered.

Skip the sunscreen. Do so for the 3 to 15 minutes prescribed to produce vitamin D for your age group (unless you're extremely sun-sensitive). A sunscreen lotion with a sun protection factor (SPF) of 8 reduces vitamin D production by 97.5 percent! If you choose to stay in the sun longer than 15 minutes, apply sunscreen (SPF 15 or higher), don sun-protective clothes, or do both. If you are fair-skinned or have an increased risk of skin cancer, you should skip sun exposure altogether and take supplemental vitamin D.

Protect your eyes. Wear good UVA/UVB sunglasses to protect your eyes from damage and increased risk of cataracts (not to mention crow's-feet).

More is not better! Don't go to tanning parlors or lie out in the sun all day long.

Fabulous Folate

Another nutrient you want to be sure to get enough of is folate. A B vitamin found in fruits and vegetables, legumes, and grains, folate is known to help prevent spinal tube birth defects, and this plus a widespread deficiency led to a federal requirement that food manufacturers start fortifying grain products with folic acid (the synthetic version of folate). In the meantime, other findings have shown that folate provides powerful protection against heart disease, colon cancer, loss of memory and mental function, and possibly Alzheimer's disease. Still, most people don't know much about folate. Here's a brief rundown of its benefits.

Homocysteine and Your Heart

Recent evidence suggests that one of the clearest markers for heart disease is a high blood level of homocysteine, an amino acid used in the building of proteins. Believed to promote the formation of arterial plaque, homocysteine is such a bad guy that people whose blood homocysteine levels are in the top 10 percent have twice the risk of heart attack and stroke as the general population. In fact, people born with a double dose of a defective gene that overproduces homocysteine are generally dead of heart disease by middle age. At this point, it's not clear whether elevated homocysteine is a cause or a consequence of heart disease. It is clear that controlling homocysteine levels is important to your health. Here's where folate is invaluable: You can lower your homocysteine levels by getting enough folate from your diet and folic acid supplements.

Unfortunately, folate in its natural form is not well absorbed by the body, and most people have a hard time getting enough of it from food. The solution is to take folic acid supplements.

The amount of folic acid found to lower homocysteine levels has ranged from 650 to 10,000 micrograms, well above the RDA of 400 micrograms. In 1998, after a USDA estimate of average daily intake of folic acid came in at 200 micrograms a day, the federal government required that folic acid be added to all enriched grain products. This initiative has had some welcome success. A follow-up study that showed the effects of fortification found an average increase in blood folate concentrations from 4.6 to 10.0 nanograms per milliliter, while homocysteine levels in the study group were slashed in half—from 18.7 to 9.8 percent.

Don't count on enriched grains, however, to take care of your full folate requirement. Few people eat enough fortified grain products to obtain the AgeLess recommendation for folate. To make the mark, focus on the folate-rich foods listed in the table "Folate" on page 252 and make up the difference with a folic acid supplement. My AgeLess recommendation is to get 800 micrograms of folate/folic acid per day from food and supplements.

The Supplement to Add at Age 55
(Now, If You're a Vegan)

Vitamin B_{12} helps to lower homocysteine levels and may preserve cognition and prevent depression. In your youth, B_{12} is abundantly available from meats, fish, and dairy products. Come the golden years, though, and even the most balanced diet may fail to yield the B_{12} you need. Why the change? Chalk it up to reduced stomach acid and hungry bacteria.

As you age, the amount of digestive acid produced by the stomach declines. This change in chemistry makes the stomach far more hospitable to digestive bacteria, which had previously limited themselves to the intestines. These hungry bacteria help to break foods down, which is good, but they also feed freely on vitamin B_{12}—which is bad.

When stomach acid levels are low, only about 1 percent of ingested vitamin B_{12} makes it past digestive bacteria and into the bloodstream. As a result, an estimated 10 to 25 percent of older Americans are deficient in vitamin B_{12}, which puts them at risk for pernicious anemia, a disease that features reduced red blood cell counts and dementia. The dementia caused by B_{12} deficiency can look a lot like Alzheimer's disease. This can cause unnecessary worry, since the deficiency can be treated but Alzheimer's can't. These days, the situation is even more complicated. Getting plenty of folate/folic acid can mask the symptoms of B_{12} deficiency, so that doctors don't detect it. And now that many foods are fortified with folic acid, doctors may be missing cases. This would be tragic since these individuals with a curable form of dementia would be treated like Alzheimer victims.

We used to treat B_{12} deficiency with injections of the vitamin to bypass stomach bacteria—but who wants those trips to the doctor and run-ins with needles? Today, we have a better way: a daily B_{12} supplement of 1 milligram (1,000 micrograms). That's 990 micrograms to satisfy the ravenous bacteria, and 10 micrograms left over to meet your body's needs.

Vegans, who eat no animal products, need to take supplemental B_{12} regardless of age. Until your 55th birthday, 10 micrograms is fine. After that, increase your dose to 1 milligram.

My AgeLess recommendation is to get 1 milligram (1,000 micrograms) of vitamin B_{12} from supplements, age 55 on.

E: Nice If You Can Get It—In Food

Finally, we come to an elusive but important nutrient in your diet: vitamin E. Eating foods containing vitamin E has consistently been shown to benefit your health and lower the risk of heart disease, and decreased dietary vitamin E can drive up your heart disease risk. The

---

HAVE AN AGELESS DAY

Nutrition

Get the Dean's Dozen foods and enjoy other life-extending delights with the following sample menu.

- **Breakfast:** Have a sliced or sectioned orange, All-Bran cereal with fat-free milk, and coffee or tea.
- **After breakfast:** Fill up your water bottle and start drinking. Take 500 milligrams of calcium.
- **Morning snack:** Drink tomato juice or crunch on baby carrots or an apple.
- **Lunch:** Try minestrone soup with tomatoes and beans and a spinach salad tossed with toasted walnuts and olive oil vinaigrette.
- **After lunch:** Take 500 milligrams of calcium.
- **Afternoon snack:** Spread peanut butter on whole wheat toast.
- **Dinner:** Serve poached salmon topped with fat-free yogurt-dill sauce, steamed broccoli drizzled with herbed olive oil, bulgar-vegetable pilaf, and a glass of red wine. Finish with fresh berries and a square of dark chocolate.
- **Shortly after dinner:** Take 500 milligrams of calcium and your vitamin D, folic acid, and vitamins B_{12} and E if you take them.

problem is, getting enough vitamin E through food can be a daunting challenge.

Found mostly in nuts and seeds, vitamin E is scarce in a normal diet. As a result, many people don't get enough. A study by the Centers for Disease Control and Prevention found that almost 30 percent of adult Americans had low blood vitamin E levels. African-Americans had the lowest, which might help explain this group's increased risk for heart disease and certain cancers. The average American diet contains about 10 milligrams of vitamin E, 66 percent of the RDA of 15 milligrams and far below the amount believed to protect against oxidative damage.

Hence the once common belief among doctors and nutritionists that vitamin E supplements could bridge the gap. But the poor performance of supplements in controlled trials suggests that buying pills could be a waste of money. So, what should you do? Even the editors of the nation's leading health newsletters are split on whether to recommend vitamin E supplements—and whether to take them themselves!

At this point, I don't believe the data supports an AgeLess recommendation to take E supplements, but chances are that a vitamin E supplement won't hurt and may help. In the meantime, my advice is to get as much vitamin E from food as you can. (See the table "Vitamin E" on page 251 for the best sources.)

The New Nutrition Rules continue to change as new information becomes available. Currently, thousands of clinical studies supported by the National Institutes of Health and other organizations are underway, and the results are likely to redefine and refine the list time and time again. I advise you to stay current with the latest recommendations at www.longevityquotient.com, and always check with your doctor before starting any vitamin, mineral, or other nutrient supplements.

Today, ask yourself: What are you going to have for lunch (or breakfast, dinner, or snack)? Will it be a fresh and natural repast replete with the nutrients that prolong life and promote great energy and looks or a high fat, processed, "convenience" food that does little more than fill you up? The choice is yours, and you have the knowledge to make it. Your longevity quotient is as good as your next meal.

YOUR AGELESS AGENDA

Nutrition

Check off each item as you achieve it:

☐ Five or more servings of fruits and vegetables a day

☐ Fish, seafood, skinless poultry, vegetable protein, pork tenderloin, or ul-tralean beef in place of high-fat red meats

☐ Monounsaturated fats (olive, canola, and nut oils) for cooking and table use instead of saturated or trans fats

☐ 250 milligrams of vitamin C from food each day

☐ Vitamin E from food—as much per day as possible

☐ 1,000 to 1,500 milligrams of calcium from food and/or through supplements each day

☐ 1,000 IU (25 milligrams) of vitamin D from food, sunlight, and/or supplements each day

☐ 800 micrograms a day of folic acid from food and/or supplements each day

☐ Two servings of fish per week

☐ Five servings of nuts per week

☐ Two to three servings of whole grains and legumes per day

☐ If you're age 55 or over, a 1,000-microgram (1-milligram) vitamin B_{12} supplement each day; 10 micrograms a day for vegans under 55

CHAPTER 3

EXERCISE

OLD EXERCISE RULE	NEW EXERCISE RULE
No pain, no gain.	**#1.** Just get off the couch.
Fitness = aerobic exercise.	**#2.** Fitness = aerobic exercise + strength training + flexibility and balance work.
Just do it.	**#3.** Put safety first.
One size fits all.	**#4.** Personalize your exercise plan.

I USED TO RACE SAILBOATS on the Chesapeake Bay. I called my sloop *Rejuvenator*—early evidence of my personal and professional goals. One of my toughest competitors was Dr. James Ricely, a cardiologist from Baltimore who sliced through the waves on a fast, dark-blue hull called *The Blue Max.* But for all his speed on the water, Jim's future looked pretty bleak from a statistical point of view. Jim suffered from type 1 diabetes (also called juvenile diabetes because it strikes in childhood). If poorly controlled, type 1 diabetes can cause blindness, kidney disease, heart and blood vessel diseases, and death. Yet today, Jim is in his mid-fifties, happily married with three children, and completely free of diabetes's deadly complications. How did Captain Jim beat not just the sailboat fleet but also the doctor's prognosis to be so healthy and fulfilled long past his probable date with disability? In addition to monitoring his blood sugar levels closely and watching his diet, Jim never misses an opportunity to exercise.

Even if you're not fighting a deadly disease, the fact holds true: No matter what your health profile, exercise can work its life-extending magic on you.

WHAT'S YOUR LONGEVITY QUOTIENT?

Exercise

To find out how your exercise habits are affecting your longevity quotient, take the following quiz. You may need to log your workouts for a week before you begin. Choose the one item from each checklist that describes you best and enter the points in the "Your LQ Points" column.

	Your LQ Points	Max LQ Points

Weekly Aerobic Exercise Time

20 points: 2 hours or more

15 points: 1 to 2 hours

10 points: 30 minutes to 1 hour

0 points: Less than 30 minutes   ____   **20**

Weekly Aerobic Exercise Level

20 points: Mostly moderate or more intense—brisk walking
        (3 to 4 miles per hour, 15- to 20-minute mile)

15 points: Mix of moderate and light activities

10 points: Mostly light—slow walking (2 to 3 miles per hour,
        20- to 30-minute mile), gardening, or housework

0 points: None   ____   **20**

Weight Training

40 points: You lift weights, use weight machines, or do
        resistance training for the eight major muscle groups
        (chest, back, abdominals, biceps, triceps, shoulders,
        buttocks/hips, legs) two times a week or more

30 points: You lift weights, use weight machines, or do resistance
        training for the eight major muscle groups once a week,
        or for a few muscle groups two times a week or more

20 points: Your daily job requires significant muscle exertion,
        but you do no other weight training

10 points: You lift weights, use weight machines, or do resistance
        training for a few muscle groups about once a week

0 points: You don't regularly lift weights, use weight
        machines, or do resistance training   ____   **40**

	Your LQ Points	Max LQ Points

Stretching and Balance Work (including stretch exercises, yoga, tai chi, Pilates, and karate)

10 points: You do some form of stretching and/or balance exercise every day of the week

8 points: You do some form of stretching and/or balance exercise most days of the week

5 points: You do some form of stretching and/or balance exercise some days of the week

3 points: You occasionally do some form of stretching and/or balance exercise

0 points: You do not do any stretching and/or balance exercise ___   **10**

Warm Up/Cool Down

5 points: You always warm up for at least 5 minutes and cool down for at least 5 minutes before and after exercise

4 points: You often warm up for at least 5 minutes and cool down for at least 5 minutes before and after exercise

3 points: You sometimes warm up for at least 5 minutes and cool down for at least 5 minutes before and after exercise

0 points: You rarely warm up for at least 5 minutes and cool ___   **5**
down for at least 5 minutes before and after exercise

Form

5 points: You've received expert instruction in weight training and stretching

3 points: You've received expert instruction in either weight training or stretching

2 points: You've read instructions about weight training and stretching

0 points: You just plunged into weight training and ___   **5**
stretching without instruction

Total   **100**

To translate your LQ score into how you're faring with the New Rules of physical fitness, find your score in the following list and read the Dean's diagnosis:

Total LQ Score	The Dean's Diagnosis
91–100	You're fit as a fiddle! Stay active and you're likely to find yourself dancing the funky chicken for many more birthdays.
81–90	Congratulations. You're getting close—but you can do better. Choose one of the AgeLess workouts as your guide to getting the right exercise mix.
71–80	You are moving around more than many Americans but not enough to optimize aging. Read this chapter to update yourself on the benefits of exercise and get started on the AgeLess workout of your choice.
61–70	You're doing something, and that beats nothing—but you're nowhere near optimal in your exercise habits, and this deficit could seriously hurt your healthspan. Get going on the AgeLess workout of your choice now.
60 or below	Full fitness alert! You're missing out on the best way to boost your health and longevity. Start the I-Don't-Have-Time-to-Exercise plan as soon as you can.

*Note: Always discuss a new exercise program with your doctor.

Exercise: Your Most Important Longevity Move

We know we *should* exercise. Yet most of us—a full 60 percent of Americans—admit that we fail to do so regularly, making a sedentary lifestyle as American as apple pie. The single most important thing you can do to ensure your physical and mental longevity is to get moving. Let me repeat that for extra emphasis: The best way to age less is to exercise.

If you believe the old rule, "no pain, no gain," that the only worthwhile exercise leaves you panting and exhausted, think again. You'll "gain" by just getting off the couch, and 30 minutes of moderate exercise a day can substantially boost your LQ.

But aerobic exercise alone is not enough. To maximize LQ, you need exercise in three complementary areas. Just as your body needs carbohydrates, protein, and fat, you need aerobic activity to condition the heart and lungs, strength training to maintain strong muscles and bones, and flexibility and balance routines to prevent injuries and falls. But as more of us are getting the exercise message, the rate of exercise-related injuries is sky rocketing. Limbering up may help keep you out of the emergency room.

Dropping out from boredom is the most common obstacle to fitness. The solution is to have more fun with your fitness plan. My Age-Less workouts let you choose your activities, exercise schedule, and exertion level while also providing the right proportion of the three types of exercise.

Exercise and the Aging Process

You need only to watch kids playing in a park to remember how natural exercise used to feel. For the young, running, jumping, dancing, and kicking are fun—pure play. My son Samuel has energy to burn. He hits the swing set every day after school not because he wants the workout, but because it feels good.

Somewhere in the teen years, though, exercise levels drop off precipitously, probably as adolescents spend more time on schoolwork and worrying about the opposite sex. For most Americans, this is the begin-

How George Beat the Grim Reaper

George Hinkle is 81. He met my coauthor, Elizabeth, at a talk she was giving to cancer survivors and came up to tell her about his own longevity "miracle." In the past 10 years, George has survived three cancer surgeries, a heart valve replacement, a staph infection in his lungs, a hip fracture, viral pneumonia, and compression fractures of two vertebrae of his spine. How did this octagenarian make it through a long list of medical threats, any one of which could have taken his life? George is a fitness buff.

George's regular routine is to walk/run 3 to 5 miles three times a week and lift weights on alternate days. After each stint in the hospital, he resumed his rehabilitation and workout schedule as soon as he could. George's doctors assured him that without his exercise habit he would no longer be here. He's not only here but recently ran and walked 81 laps, one for each year of his age (which adds up to over 20 miles), for the American Cancer Society's Relay for Life. George considers himself living proof that exercise strengthens life force not only when you're enjoying good health, but even more when illness or accidents threaten your very future.

ning of the end—the loss of exercise as play and a new perception that it's just another job.

The decline in physical activity continues into middle age; most of us settle into some kind of exercise pattern—usually at a level too low for optimum longevity. Stretching and weight training often get short shrift now, just as shrinking muscles and stiffening tendons and joints need them the most. The good news is that if you use your youthful

What to Expect When . . .

Here are some of the age-related patterns in fitness and exercise habits.

- **Teens:** Exercise now is important to obtain maximum peak bone mass—but by age 15, most teens start to seriously slack off on physical activity, perhaps distracted by the demands of schoolwork and a powerful interest in the opposite sex.
- **Twenties:** The erosion of exercise patterns continues, and many people aren't as fit at age 21 as they were at 12. Still, busy lives and high energy levels find most twentysomethings getting some exercise even if by accident.
- **Thirties and forties:** Family relationships and career consume more time, leaving us little energy and inclination to exercise. Vanity may be most people's prime motivator to exercise now, but health and longevity should be. Muscle strength peaks and begins to decline unless you counter the trend with a strength-training program. Slowing reaction times, shortening ligaments, and less-elastic tendons increase the risk of sports injuries. Proper warm up, stretching, and self-monitoring become paramount.
- **Fifties and sixties:** People who let their physical fitness level slip will start to notice difficulty in daily tasks such as getting out of chairs, lifting, and carrying. Your quality of life increasingly relies on getting regular exercise. Retirees, in their wisdom, are more likely to add flexibility and resistance work to their exercise routines, which is great for longevity—but you don't need to wait this long!
- **Seventies and eighties:** Physical fitness can make the difference between independent living and a nursing home or assisted living facility.

body, you won't lose it. Most of the changes in body shape and energy levels you start to see in your thirties are wholly preventable with a regular workout routine.

As baby boomers, the most fitness-conscious generation of Americans, celebrate bigger birthdays, they are exercising, which is terrific. But many fail to allow for the physical changes of middle age: slower reaction times, diminished joint flexibility, and less-elastic tendons. Thus, we are seeing another boom—in sports injuries. Pulled muscles, torn ligaments and tendons, dislocated joints, broken bones, and other injuries can sideline us for months and even may turn into lifelong disabilities.

Striking the right balance between enthusiasm and safety is key to exercising in middle age. And there's a double payoff to establishing good exercise habits now: You're likely to continue them through your golden years and stay fit for life. Sedentary folks will one day discover that they literally can't get off their couches even if they try.

Seventy percent or more of older Americans fail to get the exercise they need. But exercise is more important than ever now. Overall fitness is the primary determinant of independence in later years, while cardiovascular conditioning is a critical factor in preventing the heart attack that ends most people's lives. The truly good news is that it's never too late to get fit.

Research studies have found extraordinary benefits for seniors from exercise. The Honolulu Heart Program, a study of the walking habits of 71- to 93-year-old men, found that the more the participants walked each week, the less likely they were to suffer a heart attack. Make a promise to yourself to exercise. Keeping this pledge is good for your healthspan.

Exercise Efficacy

One of the uncontested facts in aging research is that people who exercise not only live longer, they live better. Here's what some important studies found:

⑥ A University of Texas study put healthy 20-year-old men in bed for 3 weeks, then let them return to their normal lives and followed them until their fiftieth birthdays. At the end of the three weeks, they were given a standard fitness test and those results were compared to the results of follow-up testing 30 years later. The eye-opening findings showed the men to be in *better* health at age 50, after living normally active lives, than they'd been after three weeks of inactivity in their prime.

◕ The Harvard Nurses' Health Study focused on the exercise habits and lifespans of 85,326 female nurses across the country over the course of 14 years. From this large, diverse group a unifying fact emerged: The more the women exercised, the longer they lived. But the improvements were by no means most dramatic for marathon runners or gym fanatics. Instead, the biggest increase in lifespan was found when women went from less than an hour per week of exercise to an average of 1 to 2 hours of weekly workout time—a seemingly slim difference with big implications. Moderately paced walking was the women's favorite form of exercise.

◕ A 22-year study of 2,014 men in midlife found that physical fitness was a strong predictor of mortality. Even small improvements in exercise habits significantly lowered the risk of death for these people in their peak productivity years.

◕ A 17-year study of people aged 60 to 94 in Alameda County, California, looked at behavioral and demographic risk factors for mortality. This seminal examination of healthy aging found a sedentary lifestyle to be a major factor in premature death (along with being overweight, smoking, skipping breakfast, and being male—sorry, guys).

◕ One of the most exciting findings of the MacArthur Foundation Study of Successful Aging was that the senior participants who

Get Married, Move Less?

Single people work out the most, which may not surprise anyone who's ever been on the body-conscious dating circuit. Married women, on the other hand, are the least active among us. I know how home life and children can complicate a schedule, but this is no reason to let your health suffer. Don't you want to be around to enjoy your golden years and play with your grandchildren?

were physically active had the best preserved mental function 10 years later. This is important evidence that a sound body and mind go hand in hand for life.

Cardiovascular Health

Exercise does wonderful things for your cardiovascular system. It conditions the heart muscle itself, lowers bad LDL cholesterol while boosting good HDL cholesterol, reduces high blood pressure, and keeps triglyceride levels in check. Regular workouts are one of the best ways to prevent heart attack and stroke, statistically the most likely causes of death for every reader of this book.

A 1999 study found that women who regularly engaged in brisk walking reduced their risk of this killer disease in the following amounts.

Hours walked per week	Coronary disease risk reduction
Less than 1	0%
1–2.9	30% (New Rule #1: The first steps provide the greatest effect!)
3–4.9	35%
5 or more	40%

As you can see, the extra time put in by the 5-hour group paid off significantly, but even the walkers at the low end of the scale upped their odds against our top killer by nearly a third.

So, I'm not talking about a trivial improvement in your longevity quotient here. Just getting off the couch will deliver a double-digit reduction in your risk of cardiovascular disease, as much as 30 percent.

People at extra risk for heart disease have even more reason to exercise, since a regular workout routine is one of your best defenses against the development and progression of this disease. The red flags for increased heart-disease risk include being male, smoking, being significantly overweight or obese (see chapter 4), and having a family history of heart attacks, high blood pressure, high cholesterol, or diabetes.

Exercise is also an important component of cardiac rehabilitation, after a heart attack, coronary artery bypass surgery, or angioplasty. Many people gain a new lease on life after these devastating events by making the fitness commitment.

Stopping Stroke

The first cousin to a heart attack (the closing of one of the coronary arteries that feeds the heart) is a stroke, which is the closing of one of the arteries that supply blood to the brain. Stroke is the nation's number three cause of death in older people. Through not always fatal, strokes can often result in permanent impairment of physical and mental functioning, making them a leading cause of disability among the elderly.

A 1999 study of 20,000 male physicians found that the doctors who managed to get one or more vigorous weekly workouts into their busy schedules had a significantly diminished risk of stroke. The greatest stroke risk reduction—19 percent—was found in the group that exercised vigorously just once a week. You don't need a lot of workout time to ward off this deadly disease.

The Nurses' Health Study tested the stroke-stopping power of exercise on 72,488 female nurses and found once again that the greatest risk reduction occurred with the first increment of exercise—between those who exercised less than 1 hour a week and those who exercised 1 to 1.9 hours a week. The risk of stroke continued to decline with additional exercise.

Cancer Prevention

Though some cancers are now treatable, prevention is clearly the preferable option. Regular exercise is known to reduce the risk of three of the deadliest cancers—breast, lung, and colon cancer—as well as pancreatic cancer, a particularly aggressive form that is almost 100 percent fatal. Consider these statistics:

- **Breast cancer:** A study following 25,000 Scandinavian women for more than a decade found that those who exercised at least 4 hours a week reduced their breast cancer risk by 33 percent— a full third.
- **Lung cancer:** In a survey of 13,905 Harvard alumni who graduated from 1916 to 1950, the inactive men were 40 percent more likely to develop lung cancer than those who did even moderate amounts of exercise.
- **Colon cancer:** The National Health and Nutrition Examination Survey (NHANES I) followed 5,138 men and 7,407 women for a decade and found that inactive individuals had a 60 percent

greater risk for colorectal cancer than participants who exercised.

⑥ **Pancreatic cancer:** Walking or hiking more than 4 hours a week
reduced the risk of pancreatic cancer, the deadliest of cancers,
by 54 percent in a large-scale study of 117,000 women and
46,000 men. Again, moderate activity was all that was required
for this protective effect.

Studies of prostate cancer, another potentially deadly cancer, are less
conclusive, but evidence suggests that exercise may lower the risk for this
type of cancer, too.

Strong Bones

You may exercise to gain strength and sculpt your muscles, but did
you know that the benefits of exercise penetrate deep into your bones,
as well? Like muscles, bones gain or maintain density with the workout
they get from weight-bearing activity. The best time to start is adolescence, when skeletal mass peaks, but exercise at any age can help bol-
ster and preserve bone mass, and so it becomes even more important as
the years go by, especially for women at risk for osteoporosis.

Brain Power

New findings in neuroscience could turn the old stereotype of the
dumb jock on its head: We now have evidence that suggests that exercise not only helps build muscles, it can multiply brain cells, too.

The once well-entrenched idea that we're born with all the brain
cells we'll ever get has been immolated by the landmark discovery that
neurogenesis, or the production of new brain cells and connections between them, continues throughout adult life. This good news was first
noted by neuroscientist Fred Gage at the Salk Institute in California.
The result has been a profound change in how scientists view the brain.
The race is on to uncover what triggers neurogenesis, and it looks like
several important factors figure in: mental and physical stimulation and
the reduction of stress, which can kill brain cells. Exercise provides both
stimulation and stress reduction.

Following in Gage's footsteps, Salk researcher Henriette van Praag
found in 2001 that adult rats who worked out on a running wheel were
creating new brain cells at a rate astonishingly higher than their seden-

tary friends. (This led to a rash of lunchtime walks among the lab's personnel.) While it's harder to study brain cell response to exercise in humans, evidence does show that physical exercise can improve people's performance on various mental tasks. That morning workout may give you an edge on the competition at work.

Exercise looks to be even more important to the brain in later life, when physical fitness provides powerful protection against dementia and Alzheimer's disease. One of the highlights of my work on the MacArthur Foundation Study of Successful Aging was discovering that the participants who exercised the most had the best mental function 10 years down the road. This was a great leap forward in our understanding of the role that physical fitness plays in successful aging. And a recent study of more than 6,000 Canadian seniors concluded that exercise of any sort keeps brain function youthful, while the highest levels of exercise can cut the incidence of cognitive impairment and dementia by up to half and of Alzheimer's by as much as 60 percent. Flex your mental muscle!

Stress Relief

From daily pressures to life-changing events, modern life is highly stressful, with real consequences for your health. (See chapter 6 for more about the damaging effect of stress.) While organization and planning are good stress reducers—it's always a good idea to prepare for that big meeting, allow extra commute time for traffic, and make checklists to pull off your daughter's wedding hitch-free—one of the best ways to manage stress is a regular exercise regimen. By relaxing muscular and mental tension, exercise controls stress hormone levels and improves both your energy and your sleep. For this reason alone, exercise belongs on your to-do list. Or think of it this way: Not exercising is not an option. No matter how busy your schedule, you will *always* accomplish more if you take the time to exercise. (See chapter 5 for more about the importance of a good night's sleep to your long, healthy life.)

Diabetes Prevention and Control

The rate of adult-onset or type 2 diabetes, a serious lifestyle-related disease marked by the inability of the body to use insulin effectively, is rising so fast that public health officials have declared it a national epidemic. With age and added pounds, our ability to convert blood sugar into energy can decline, leading to a condition known as insulin resistance. Face this change passively, and your risk of type 2 diabetes increases dramatically. Get active, and you can make great strides toward preventing diabetes or managing the condition if you have it.

Experts consider exercise and diet the most important preventive measures you can take against diabetes. For one thing, diet and exercise work together to reduce excess weight, a major risk factor for type 2 diabetes. Furthermore, the muscle contractions required by exercise remove sugar from the bloodstream, stabilizing blood sugar levels and helping to prevent development of insulin resistance. For people with diabetes, getting physically fit and losing a few pounds can reduce or even eliminate the need for insulin and other medications to control blood sugar.

Arthritis Relief

Osteoarthritis, the painful stiffening of joints from age or overuse, will hit us all if we live long enough. Rheumatoid arthritis, an autoimmune disease with similar though often more crippling symptoms, can strike at any time. For sufferers of either type of arthritis, movement is so difficult that the idea of exercising seems completely counterintuitive—however, a number of studies have shown that exercise can actually reduce pain and improve the function of diseased joints. No one knows how it works, but it does.

Independence

When asked about their greatest concerns about aging, most people don't give the answer you'd expect. We fear disability far more than we fear death, and our fear is not unfounded. By the time you reach age 85, as most baby boomers will, there's a 50 percent chance that you'll need help in such daily tasks as bathing, dressing, walking, preparing meals, shopping, or even going to the toilet. We dread the idea of ending up in a nursing home, and few of us have family members who can be full-time caregivers or the resources to afford private home health or nursing home care. How do we save ourselves from this "fate worse than death"? The answer (it's a no-brainer) is regular exercise.

The first challenge is to stay strong enough to get in and out of chairs, bed, and the bathtub unassisted. The next is to stay on your feet once you get there. Falls are a leading cause of permanent disability and even death in older people. A third of the 65-plus population takes a spill each year, making falls the most common cause of injury in this age group. Half of 80- to 89-year-olds fall at least once a year. As you age, frail hipbones are more likely to break in a fall—it happens to some 300,000 Americans annually—and 20 percent of those who suffer a hip fracture die within 12 months. For survivors, the chances of winding up in a nursing home increase more than five times over.

How does exercise help keep you on your feet? By toning muscles, improving posture, training the body to transfer weight, and extending your range of motion, a fitness routine can help you continue to move gracefully for the years to come. Many types of exercise support active aging; as an example consider tai chi, a type of balance training that's great for improving balance and reducing the fear of falling. Walking is also a winner. A study of 9,516 women found that those who walked regularly reduced their risk of hip fracture by 30 percent, with protection increasing with the distance covered. Another clinical trial determined that men and women who engaged in 2 to 4 hours a week of moderate activity such as walking, biking, light housekeeping, or gardening trimmed their hip fracture risk by 28 percent.

NEW EXERCISE RULE #1:
JUST GET OFF THE COUCH

Exercise is an amazing elixir of youth. The problem is, we don't do it. Look around you. Three out of four people aren't getting the basic government recommendation for exercise—30 minutes, most days of the week. One in four never exercises at all. Are you one of them?

The Birth of the Couch Potato

Once upon a time, unless you were very rich, life was full of physical activity. Transportation consisted of your own two feet, or if you were lucky you rode a horse. Farming was the main occupation and required hard manual labor from dawn to dusk. Without modern "labor-saving" devices, washing, cooking, cleaning, and shopping were all serious workouts. Wealthy folks who had the luxury of avoiding such exertions turned up their noses at such labors, getting their workouts at the occasional formal dance or fox hunt but considering sweat as déclassé as dirty hands.

The Industrial Revolution radically changed our occupations and lifestyles. Machines started doing the hard jobs, at work and at home, and when radio, television, movies, and computers came along to fill the extra free time, we were only too happy to take a seat and a load off our feet. So our couch potato culture was born—a 20th-century phenomenon that is proving to be one of the greatest public health threats of the modern age.

Being a couch potato can create a vicious cycle, since being sedentary leaves you short on energy and verve. A variety of excuses keep you sitting down. I don't have time. The gym is too far away. Gee, the weather looks nasty. I don't have a workout buddy. Here's the most insidious: I'll never have a perfect body, so why bother?

No More Excuses: Move for Just 30 Minutes a Day

Our couch potato problem may not come from a collective decision to go to pot so much as from the famous all-or-nothing American attitude. Many people think that workouts without blood, sweat, and tears are worthless—so forget about it.

In 1995, the country's leading health experts announced that this thinking was scientifically all wrong. On the contrary, the latest evidence shows that just 30 minutes of moderate movement a day can make the difference. An adequate workout doesn't have to be painful or hard.

Like saving for retirement, it's far more important that you get in a little *regular* exercise than that you try to break any records. Despite

Sweat Less

In 1995, the American College of Sports Medicine changed its recommendation for exercise from *hard* workouts, 3 days per week, in 20- to 30-minute sessions to *moderate* workouts, 5 to 7 days per week, in sessions that add up to 30 minutes per day. Each session can be as short as 8 minutes long.

what your past gym teachers or coaches might have shouted from the sidelines, there's no failing grade for exercise other than failing to exercise at all. In fact, in 1995 the American College of Sports Medicine lowered its minimum recommended exercise intensity level from 60 percent to 50 percent of your maximum heart rate. What's more, you don't have to do it all at once. Short exercise sessions are just as beneficial as long ones, as long as you get at least 30 minutes' worth each day. Small choices like walking up stairs instead of taking the elevator add up to big health gains when done regularly.

By the way, fitness buffs will be happy to hear that you can get additional benefits by working out a little longer and harder: Raising

A Tale of Two Generations

Here's a story that shows how the conveniences of modern living can sap vitality from our later years. My grandmother, Mindla Soskin, or Minnie as everyone called her, lived to be 89 and spent a grand total of 1 day of her life in a hospital. Sure, she spent time in a nursing home during her eighties, but she was only there as a visiting volunteer assisting those "older persons" who could no longer fend for themselves. My mom, Ann, on the other hand, turned 89 in a nursing home, not as a volunteer but as a resident. Mom and Minnie were about the same height and weight, didn't smoke or drink, and shared the same diet and other habits. The big difference between them was their activity levels.

While Minnie walked, climbed stairs, carried groceries, and cleaned her house every day, Mom drove her car everywhere, took the elevator instead of stairs, and had help with the heavy household cleaning. Without a supplementary exercise program, these "conveniences" took a high toll on Mom's healthspan. She's now suffered four hip fractures (yes, though you only have two hips you can break them more than once), and she can no longer walk.

Sadly, Mom and Minnie's story shows the serious backward progress our society is making in physical fitness. The moral of this story of two Jewish grandmothers is that Minnie's significant fitness advantage was gained without long, sweaty hours at the gym. She never visited one! Simple daily activities kept Minnie on her feet, and you can likewise design a more active lifestyle, even in the deskbound information age.

your heart rate as high as 75 percent of your maximum and extending your workout sessions to 60 minutes 5 or more days a week can increase your gain.

FITNESS = AEROBIC EXERCISE + STRENGTH TRAINING + FLEXIBILITY AND BALANCE WORK

Though you don't have to knock yourself out to exercise for longevity, you do need the right mix of activities. Be sure to get aerobic exercise to condition the cardiovascular system, strength training to maintain strong muscles and bones, and a flexibility and balance program for strength and flexibility.

Aerobic Exercise for a Healthy Heart and Arteries

Aerobic activity, the vigorous movement that raises heart rate, can keep your cardiovascular system young to ward off heart attacks or related cardiovascular conditions. This is no small benefit when you consider these events are the leading cause of mortality in the U.S. Aerobic exercise can also burn calories to support your lithe figure and blithe spirit, lower your blood pressure, improve your metabolism of sugar, enhance sleep, and boost your mood. An aerobic workout can be as easy as walking with friends; just keep up a lively pace and don't shy away from hills. An 18-hole golf game does the job if you leave the cart at the clubhouse; salsa dancers get to count their nights out on the dance floor.

NEW RULES FOR SMOKERS
Fitness

If you smoke and haven't yet been able to quit, exercise is one of the best ways to reduce your chances of getting lung cancer or heart disease. And who knows? The psychological boost you get from feeling fit might help you kick the habit.

Aerobics Beats Genetics

One aspect of the MacArthur Foundation Study of Successful Aging looked at how twins fared in relation to their aerobic exercise habits. Aerobics blew genetics away. Individuals who walked briskly or jogged for 30 minutes just *six times a month* had a *40 percent lower* risk of dying than their twins who did not exercise. So take heart if you come from a family with a history of cardiovascular disease or other killer illnesses. Regular aerobic exercise (and other AgeLess habits) can outweigh your genetic endowment.

Choose from these aerobic activities for your AgeLess workout.

Light	Moderate	Vigorous
Ballroom dancing	Badminton	Aerobic or step dancing
Croquet	Bicycling (easy)	Backpacking
Fishing (stream and lake)	Bowling	Basketball
	Calisthenics	Bicycling (fast)
Gardening (raking, weeding)	Car washing	Exercise machines (treadmill, stairclimber, stationary bicycles, rowing machine, elliptical trainer, etc.)
Pool exercises (gentle)	Fishing (deep sea)	Gardening (digging, hand mowing)
Sailing (large boats)	Gardening (hedging or planting seedlings)	Jogging
Walking (2 mph)	Golf	Jumping rope
	Housework	Power walking (faster than 3 mph)
	Hunting	Racquetball
	Ping-Pong	Roller skating or blading
	Pool exercises (more intense)	Running
	Snorkeling	Scuba diving
	Softball	Skiing
	Surfing	Soccer
	Walking (3 mph)	Lap swimming
		Tennis
		Volleyball

For building bone mass—an AgeLess goal—weight-bearing exercise is best. Swimming doesn't strengthen your bones as efficiently as exercise in which you support your own weight. (Some people with arthritis or other conditions rely on water's buoyancy to make their workout comfortable, which is fine.)

KATHY SMITH'S

Top 10 Power Walking Tips

One of the first fitness experts to promote the benefits of walking workouts, Kathy Smith has been helping people step out successfully for years. Here are her top 10 power walking tips:

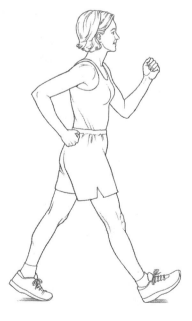

1. **Feet first.** Wear high-quality walking shoes and absorbent socks.
2. **Dress right.** Wear layers that you can take off as you warm up.
3. **Start slow.** Begin your walk at an easy to moderate speed to warm up, then stop for some stretches if you plan to push the pace or do intervals.
4. **Work from the core.** Focus on using your core—the abdominal muscles—to initiate the stride and stabilize your torso.
5. **Focus on posture.** Keep your head and neck elongated, chest open, collarbones wide, shoulder blades down, and spine straight.
6. **Swing.** Drive the arms to speed the legs.
7. **Shorten.** As you build up speed, shorten your stride so your legs can go faster.
8. **Climb.** Include hills in your walking terrain at least once a week.
9. **Push.** Twice a week, add bursts of speed, or intervals, to your walk. Depending on your condition, start with 15- to 30-second intervals, recovering for 1 minute after each one and repeating 4 to 5 times. Work up to 5 to 10 intervals each lasting 1 to 2 minutes, with 1 minute recovery in between.
10. **Stretch.** Always stretch after a power walk.

For more walking wisdom from Kathy, see her book *Kathy Smith's Walkfit for a Better Body* (Warner Books).

Exercise Machines: Excuse Eliminators

One great way to overcome exercise excuses is to buy a "cardio" exercise machine (treadmill, stairclimber, stationary bike, elliptical trainer, rower, or ski machine) or join a gym that has one or more you like. Whatever the weather or your current energy level, cardio equipment enables you to work out indoors at the level of your choice, often providing gadgets to keep you amused as you go.

The upside of exercise machines is that you don't have to worry about the weather. The downside is monotony: flat-out boredom. You may find that staring at the same familiar wall for 30 minutes every day gets old fast—so enhance your exercise with entertainment. Place a television facing your equipment (VCR, DVD, ReplayTV, or TiVo optional), and watch your favorite programs while you walk, run, or row. Install stereo speakers to either side of your equipment and find your groove with music. Take a portable tape or CD player to the gym. If you like to read while you work out, look for equipment with a rack to hold a magazine or book. A nearby window can also improve your exercise environment with natural light, scenery, and fresh air.

Treadmill Tips

Among cardio machines, exercise physiologists tend to favor the treadmill, and I like them, too, because they allow you to walk—the safest and most popular exercise—regardless of the weather. Here are some pointers for choosing and using your equipment.

- Look for a little padding on the track and easy, quick adjustment of incline level and speed.
- Get a safety connection that attaches to your body and turns the machine off immediately if you stumble or fall—an increasingly important protection as you age and your risk of falls and serious injury increases. Use it. It could be a lifesaver.
- Try a speed of 3 to 4 miles per hour with a slight incline of 5 percent to reach your target exertion rate.
- If you have extra money to spend, consider higher-priced models that calculate calories expended, monitor your heart rate, and more.

Fitness

MYTH

Running killed Jim Fixx.

FACT

Jim Fixx, the man who brought marathons to the masses in the 1970s, seemed to fall victim to his own prescription when he died at age 52 while midstride on a run. Some people tried to use Fixx's tragic death as an argument against vigorous aerobic activity, but in fact his exercise habit probably bought him an extra decade of life. Fixx, whose father died of a heart attack at age 43, had serious heart disease, high cholesterol, and chest pains that he never treated, as well as a former smoking habit. Exercise can extend and improve your life, but it can't substitute for medical attention to serious disease.

Strength Training for Muscle and Bone Mass

Contrary to popular misconception, it's never too late to start weight training. Building and preserving muscle mass is important to a great appearance now and independence in your later years. For most people, muscle size and strength peaks during the twenties or thirties and then starts the downward slide that eventually makes it tough to get out of the bathtub, rise from an easy chair, pick up a grandchild, or carry a bag of groceries. But this decline is not inevitable! Scientists have been looking long and hard for the enzyme, gene, or other biological factor that causes loss of muscle mass with age. Fortunately for

Try Secondhand Equipment

As New Year's resolutions fade, you're likely to find used treadmills, barbells, and other home exercise equipment at garage sales, listed in the classifieds, or on the Internet at bargain prices. Though sad for the lapsed exercisers, don't hesitate to let one person's loss be your gain. You can outfit your home gym at a reasonable price and have enough money left to buy some new workout clothes.

us, the results all point to a different cause: behavior. As the years go by, people use their muscles less, and the use-it-or-lose-it principle kicks in to shrink your biceps and soften your buns of steel. The solution is strength training.

Strength training is not just for people who aspire to look like Arnold Schwarzenegger! Strong muscles come in many shapes and sizes. You don't have to add bulk while you gain strength; in fact, lifting weights can burn fat to trim and tone you in all the right places. Pumping iron, pulling resistance bands, and doing isometrics (exercises against the weight of your body) all offer effective prevention of many diseases and disorders along with a nice cosmetic payoff.

Use dumbbells to ease depression. When you're feeling down, you might want to try picking up a couple of dumbbells. A study out of Harvard Medical School has shown that a progressive resistance training program can be an effective antidepressant. Working out with weights releases endorphins, brain hormones that improve your sense of well-being. Comments about your new firmer muscles can also make you feel better!

Prevent and recover from injury. Weight training can also help counter past mistakes and prevent future ones. I know this principle by personal experience. I started skiing in my teens, years before the introduction of safety bindings. To get the best performance from the wooden skis and leather boots we used then, we tied our boots directly to the skis with straps called Long Thongs. I entered my first and last downhill race with these Long Thongs tied as tight as I could get them. At the second gate, I caught a ski edge in the snow, and according to eyewitness accounts, did a two-and-a-half gainer in the air (unintentional and zero points for style) before returning to earth with my skis going in two different directions and my body in a third. My penalty was a torn cartilage and a ripped ligament in my left knee.

Torn knee cartilage and ligaments are among the most common injuries in a variety of sports, including skiing, basketball, and football. I continued to ski, but I unconsciously favored my weakened knee. For the next decade, my skiing became progressively worse. I was about ready to throw in the towel on one of my favorite pastimes when an orthopedic surgeon suggested that I start a weight-training program to build up the muscles around my knee joint. He also suggested that I wear a brace while skiing to protect my knee against any twisting motions that might cause further injury. Between the strength exercises and the brace I returned to my old self on the slopes. I'm still at it in my sixties—along with windsurfing and singles tennis.

Shoulder injuries are also common, especially among baseball pitchers, tennis players, and golfers. Rotator cuff injuries affect tendons of the muscles that insert into the shoulder. Bursitis, the inflammation of the shoulder joint lining, is another frequent complaint. I managed to sustain a rotator cuff injury from skiing, too. Fortunately, the same principle held as for my knee. Building up the muscles around the shoulder both reduced my pain and allowed me to avoid corrective surgery. Strengthening your muscles helps you to get active again, boosting your healthspan—and strong muscles can prevent sports injuries in the future.

Live more independently. By your seventies and eighties, physical strength is central to your quality of life. Your ability to accomplish the simple daily tasks I mentioned before—getting in and out of an armchair or the bathtub, shopping, cooking, getting dressed—ultimately define the difference between independence and relying on a caregiver's help.

Fortunately, we never lose our ability to buff up the muscles that support independent living. For instance, researchers from Tufts University got great results from weight training in a group of 80- and 90-year-old residents at a Boston area nursing home. They started some of the seniors on a weight-lifting program and the rest on nutritional supplements without strength training. The weight-training group followed a regimen of progressive resistance training of the hip and knee extensors, 3 days a week for 10 weeks. Muscle strength increased by over 100 percent in those in the strength-training group. Furthermore, their walking speed increased 12 percent and their ability to climb stairs by 28 percent. The weight trainers had more spontaneous activity and their thigh-muscle area increased significantly, while the control group lost muscle mass. A year later, the scientists found that the weight-training group not only outsurvived the sedentary supplement group but also had better health. Many of them were walking with minimal assistance for the first time in years.

No matter what your age, the time to start strength training is now.

Strength-Training Basics

Here are some ground rules for getting started on your strength-training program.

⑥ **Get professional guidance.** Weight training is a powerful type of exercise that presents a significant risk of muscle strain or joint injury if you don't use proper form. The first step for safe strength training is to get some professional instruction, whether from a group class, a personal trainer, or a staff member at a gym.

⑥ **Choose your equipment.** If you belong to a gym, explore the weight machines, which help guide your form and range of motion. Handheld or strap-on weights are affordable and easy to use at home or the office. Resistance bands, elastic cords that provide resistance as you pull them taut, are even more portable; try packing them in your luggage when you travel. Isometric exercises require only the weight of your body—an anytime, anywhere strength-training option.

⑥ **Set your goals.** Are you interested in building up muscle (actually seeing those biceps grow), slightly increasing muscle size and contour, or simply gaining strength and muscle tone? Achieving any of these goals can improve your LQ. Simply choose your weights, set length, and progression strategy in accord with your objectives.

Goal	Set Length *Choose the heaviest weight you can lift for:*	Progression Strategy *Increase weight as muscle strength grows?*
To build muscle	6–8 repetitions	Yes
To slightly increase muscle size and definition	8–12 repetitions	Yes, slowly
The Dean's Choice: To gain strength and tone without building size	15–20 repetitions	No

⑥ **Do one set per muscle group.** Most of the benefits of strength training—as much as 80 percent or more—are attained in the first set, so you can maximize your time investment by doing a single set of each exercise, then moving on to the next muscle group.

⑥ **Cover all eight muscle groups.** The single-set strategy helps ensure you get to all the eight major muscle groups with each workout session. Do one set apiece for each of the following: chest, back, abdominals, biceps, triceps, shoulders, buttocks/hips, and legs.

⑥ **Raise your heart rate.** You can keep your heart rate elevated throughout your strength-training session by starting with a vigorous warmup (or your aerobic workout), keeping your movements brisk, and proceeding directly to the next exercise without rest. Working out in this zone helps to burn fat and condition your cardiovascular system.

⑥ **Do your workout every other day.** A day off between strength-training sessions allows your muscles to rest and revitalize.

KATHY SMITH'S

Top 10 Home Strength-Training Exercises

Want to boost metabolism, build stronger bones, and sculpt your body? Kathy Smith says train for strength. Here are her favorite exercises to do at home. All you need are a pair of dumbbells, a sturdy chair, a stair or platform, and a pillow. Use dumbbell weights that you can comfortably lift for 6 to 20 repetitions, according to your training goal. The weight will depend on your strength and the particular exercise.

CHEST

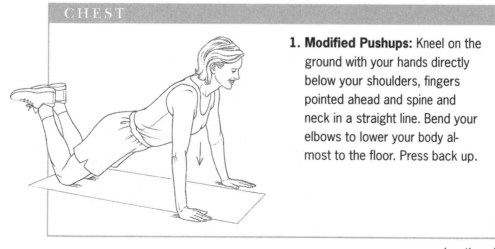

1. Modified Pushups: Kneel on the ground with your hands directly below your shoulders, fingers pointed ahead and spine and neck in a straight line. Bend your elbows to lower your body almost to the floor. Press back up.

(continued)

KATHY SMITH'S *Top 10 Home Strength-Training Exercises (cont.)*

BACK

2. Bent-Over Rows: Sit in a chair with a pillow in your lap and dumbbells in your hands. Lean forward to rest your chest on the pillow. Lift your elbows up and out to the sides until in line with your shoulders, palms facing to the back. Lower down to your starting position.

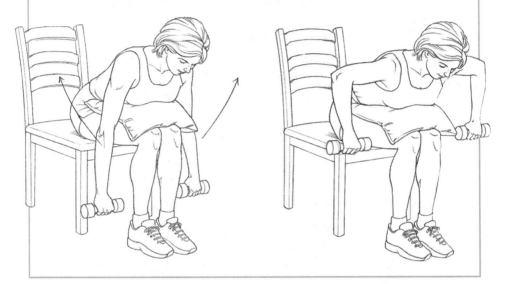

BACK

3. Back Extensions: Lie on your stomach, tops of your feet to the floor and your forehead resting on your hands with your elbows out to the side. Keeping your feet on the floor, lift your head, hands, and chest as high as you comfortably can. Return to the starting position.

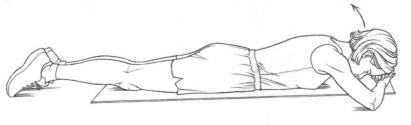

ABDOMINALS

4. Abdominal Curl-Ups: Lie on your back with knees bent and feet flat on the floor. Place your hands behind your head, elbows out to the side. Lift your head, neck, and rib cage a few inches off the floor, tightening your abdominals and tucking your pelvis under. Return. Do not pull on your neck during the exercise. To avoid neck strain, keep your chin forward.

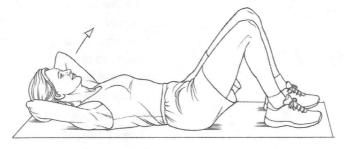

BICEPS

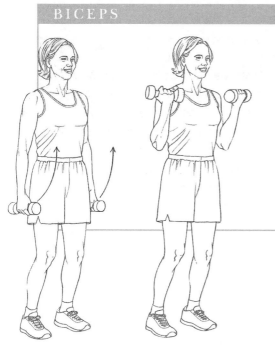

5. Biceps Curls: Stand with your feet shoulder-width apart and knees slightly bent, arms hanging at your side with a dumbbell in each hand. Curl the dumbbells up toward your shoulders, rotating them out to face the back and be slightly wider than your elbows. Lower back down.

(continued)

KATHY SMITH'S *Top 10 Home Strength-Training Exercises (cont.)*

TRICEPS

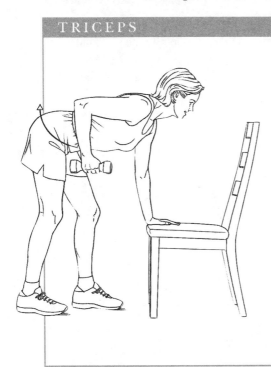

6. Triceps Kickbacks: Stand in front of a chair with your left foot slightly in front of your right foot and a dumbbell in your right hand. Bend your legs slightly and bend at the hips, keeping your back straight, to place your left hand on the seat of the chair. Bend and lift your right elbow until it's slightly higher than your body, your palm facing in. Holding your elbow in place, straighten your arm to the back until the arm is straight and the dumbbell points toward the floor. Return to the starting position. Repeat on the other side.

SHOULDERS

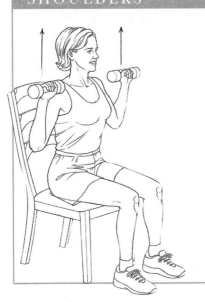

7. Overhead Presses: Sit in a chair with a dumbbell in each hand, back straight and feet flat on the floor. Place your hands at shoulder level, elbows bent and palms facing forward. Raise the dumbbells upward and slightly in front of your head until your arms are straight. Return.

SHOULDERS

8. Side Lateral Raises: Holding dumbbells, stand with your feet at shoulder width and knees slightly bent. Raise your arms straight out to the sides with your palms facing down until your hands are slightly higher than your shoulders. Return.

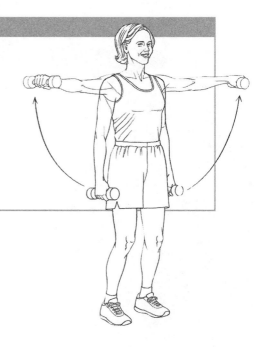

BUTTOCKS AND HIPS

9. Chair Stand and Reverse Chair Stand: Start seated in a chair. Stand up, without using your arms if possible. For the reverse, sit back down, again without arms if you can.

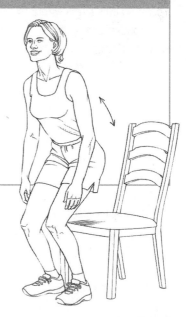

(continued)

KATHY SMITH'S *Top 10 Home Strength-Training Exercises (cont.)*

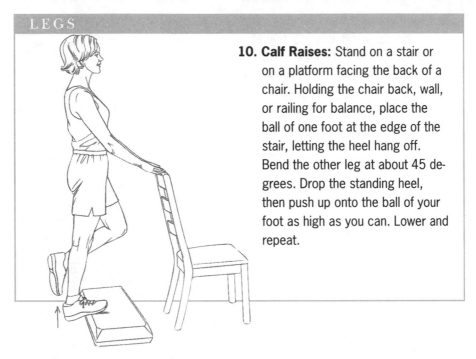

LEGS

10. Calf Raises: Stand on a stair or on a platform facing the back of a chair. Holding the chair back, wall, or railing for balance, place the ball of one foot at the edge of the stair, letting the heel hang off. Bend the other leg at about 45 degrees. Drop the standing heel, then push up onto the ball of your foot as high as you can. Lower and repeat.

You can find Kathy's complete 12-week strength training program in her book *Kathy Smith's Lift Weights to Lose Weight* (Warner Books). Women in or approaching menopause can also find guidance in *Kathy Smith's Moving through Menopause* (Warner Books).

Flexibility and Balance Work

For 10 years, I was involved in developing a new research center in Marin County, California, called the Buck Institute on Aging. Marin County is considered an epicenter of health consciousness, and we thought it was the ideal setting for a laboratory to study future health trends in the general population. An interesting discovery we made at the Buck Institute was that the most common cause of disability in Marin seniors aged 85 and older was problems with balance. This study suggests that imbalance-related falls may become the number-one cause of disability in health-conscious baby boomers when they reach their eighties, ahead of arthritis, heart disease, and dementia.

Stretch for suppleness and strength. Stretching offers several benefits for your AgeLess body. Besides releasing muscle tension and improving posture, stretching can also protect against injury—both the
falls I just mentioned and the aches, pains, and accidents that can arise
in an active lifestyle. Supple muscles and elastic tendons are less likely
to get torn or suffer spasms as you chase a tennis ball or attempt a high
kick in aerobics class. Stretching also strengthens lower-back muscles,
minimizing back problems. Finally, stretching after exercise prevents
soreness so you can get back at it again tomorrow.

A daily stretch is just what the doctor ordered to stay flexible and in-
jury-free. To get the maximum benefit, stretch after you've warmed up
with some light activity to loosen the muscles and increase blood flow. Also
be sure to stretch the muscles you've worked after each exercise session.

Practice balance postures. Stretching improves your balance overall,
but there are also specific exercises you can do that improve *propriocep-
tion*, what physiologists call our inner perception of our body's orienta-
tion. A complex balancing act governed by the inner ear keeps us
upright, and you can fine-tune this ability by practicing balance postures.

The ancient martial art of tai chi is one such system. Tai chi is meant
to maintain balance of your *chi*, or life energy—and along the way this
workout can also improve your balance, tone muscles, lower blood pressure, ease the pain of arthritis, and reduce stress. Deep breathing helps
you relax and focus your attention on slow, dancelike movements that
reflect the rhythms of nature. Each arm or leg motion is countered with
one in the opposite direction, providing a complete workout while
bringing chi into harmony and balance. If your goal is mastery, tai chi
can be a demanding discipline even for accomplished athletes, and yet
almost anyone can benefit. Whether you're a thirtysomething looking
for a new challenge or 80-plus in search of a workout that's nice to your
joints and helps prevent falls, tai chi is an exercise you can continue for
a lifetime.

Opportunities to learn and practice tai chi range from community
groups practicing out in the park to health clubs, studios, and college
extension courses. After some hands-on instruction, you may also want
to explore books and tapes on the subject.

Several other systems offer stretching and balance training. Pilates uses
slow exercises that target stomach and back muscles to strengthen your

"core." Known for shaping long, lean muscles, Pilates can be done on a mat or on a specially designed machine with ropes and pulleys to guide your movements. Yoga, the Indian system of held postures, is offered as a class at many health clubs and studios and is easy to do at home. Karate is a martial art with a focus on combat. Faster and more vigorous than tai chi, karate combines the benefits of balance, stretch, and cardiovascular exercise.

KATHY SMITH'S

Top 10 Stretches

Kathy Smith insists that we can actually become *more* flexible as we grow older. All you have to do is stretch. Here are her stretching picks:

Try to hold each stretch for at least 10 to 30 seconds, gradually increasing your time as you gain flexibility. Don't strain, and never stretch to the point where you feel pain.

1. **Quad/Hip Flexor Stretch:** Stand facing the back of a chair and hold the chair's back with your left hand for balance. Bend your right knee and raise your foot behind you, holding it with your right hand and gently pushing your heel toward your buttocks. Repeat with the other leg.

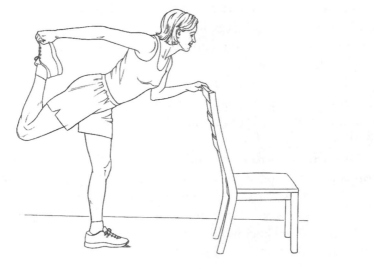

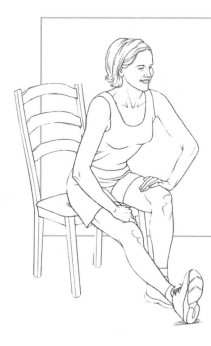

2. Hamstring/Calf Stretch: Sit on the edge of a chair with your left leg bent and your right leg extended in front of you. Place your hands on your thighs, flex the right foot, and lean forward from the hips until you feel the stretch. Repeat on the other side.

3. Supine Spine Twist: Lie on your back with your legs outstretched. Pull your right knee to your chest, pausing a moment to feel the stretch. Extend your right arm straight out to the side and with your left hand, gently pull the right knee across the body and toward the floor on the other side. Keep both shoulders on the ground. Return and repeat on the other side.

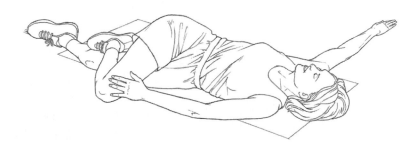

(continued)

KATHY SMITH'S *Top 10 Stretches (cont.)*

4. Extended Child's Pose: Kneel on the floor with knees hip-width apart. Sit down on your heels and bring your chest down to your thighs, resting your forehead on the floor and extending your arms straight overhead.

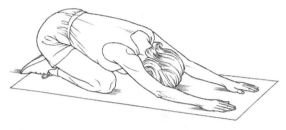

5. Triceps Stretch: Place your left hand at the base of your neck, moving your elbow as high as you can with your forearm and upper arm close to your ear. Press the elbow back with your right hand to feel a stretch in the triceps.

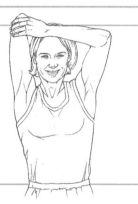

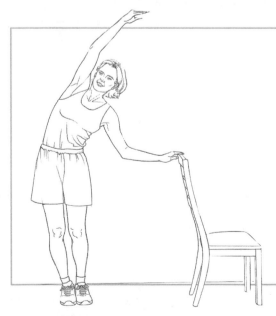

6. Outer Hip/Torso Stretch: Stand sideways to the back of a chair with your feet together and your left hand resting on the chair back for balance. Extend your right arm over your head and bend as far as you can to the left, reaching to feel the stretch. Turn around and repeat on the other side.

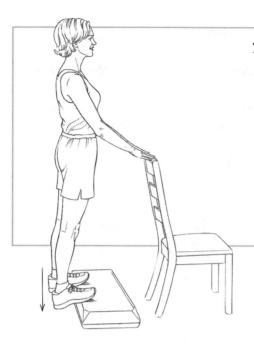

7. Calf Stretch: Stand with the balls of your feet on the edge of a platform or stair. Hold on to the chair or wall for balance. Lower your heels until you feel a stretch in your calves. For a deeper stretch, try one leg at a time.

8. Modified Cobra: Lie face down on the floor. Place your palms in front of you on the floor near shoulder level and press your upper body up, keeping your pubic bone on the floor. Go as high as you comfortably can, keeping your elbows bent and close to your body.

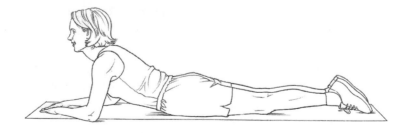

(continued)

KATHY SMITH'S *Top 10 Stretches (cont.)*

9. Standing Cat Back/Abdominal Stretch: Stand facing the front of a chair. Slightly bend your knees and bend forward to place your palms flat on the chair seat. Lift your head and push your hips away to arch your back. Reverse, pulling in your abdominals, dropping your head, and rounding your back toward the ceiling.

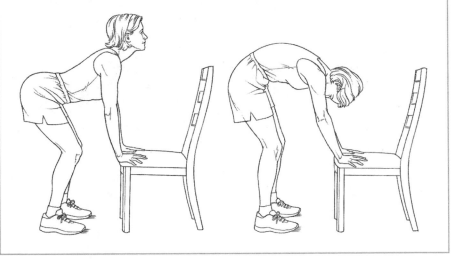

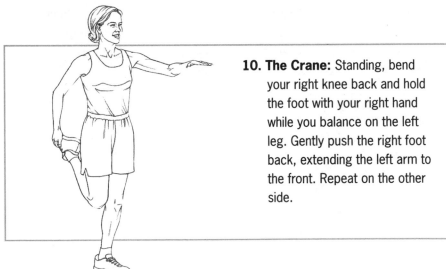

10. The Crane: Standing, bend your right knee back and hold the foot with your right hand while you balance on the left leg. Gently push the right foot back, extending the left arm to the front. Repeat on the other side.

For more about stretching from a Smith point of view, see *Kathy Smith's Lift Weights to Lose Weight* (Warner Books).

PUT SAFETY FIRST

Michigan, fall of 1998: Four men die while hunting deer—not by stray bullets, but from heart attacks. Two of the fallen were found next to the dead deer they were trying to drag to their vehicles.

Sudden strenuous effort in an otherwise sedentary lifestyle can at best give you sore or strained muscles, and you don't have to be hunting in the Michigan woods to be vulnerable. Worse, it can lead to the kinds of falls and injuries I've been talking about. Worst of all, many Americans from Buffalo to Boise die each year while shoveling their driveways after the first snowstorm of the year, gunning their hearts into overdrive with no warm up.

People exercising improperly or beyond their abilities are also more likely to suffer from run-of-the-mill injuries in the course of exercise. Sports injuries are on the rise in the aging population, and this trend could counteract the benefits of an active lifestyle if left unchecked. From 1990 to 1996, sports-related injuries to 65-year-olds increased by 54 percent, while seniors riding bicycles saw their injury rate rise 75 percent. Among the estimated 11,000 emergency-room visits by bicycling seniors in 1996 were countless head injuries that could have been prevented by wearing a helmet.

To exercise in your safety zone, it is essential that you follow these AgeLess principles:

- Start your exercise program slowly and gradually increase your level.
- Warm up for 5 minutes before you begin all-out exercise and take 5 minutes to cool down, gradually decreasing the intensity of exercise until your breathing returns to normal.
- Stretch at the end of every workout.
- Wear appropriate protective gear (helmets, kneepads, etc.).
- Get professional instruction in correct form for any new exercise, especially lifting weights and using equipment. The number of emergency-room visitors injured using exercise equipment and lifting weights rose 173 percent from 1990 to 1996. Though books and videos can help you learn about proper form, live instruction offers precise personalized feedback.

Running Increases Injury Risk

Though running is a powerful cardiovascular conditioner, it carries a sizable risk of injury. One study found that 35 to 65 percent of runners are injured each year, with the likelihood of a musculoskeletal mishap increasing with the weekly distance run. If you run, wear good shoes, run on evenly graded ground, and seek out softer surfaces. Warm up before every run. If you start to feel tired, walk.

◎ Don't follow 5 days at your desk with a long, sweaty basketball game or 8 hours on the slopes. Build exercise into your weekday routine to avoid weekend-warrior risks, and remember that doing a little all or most days of the week is far better than waiting until you think you have time.

Exercising with Arthritis

Exercise is one of the best therapies for arthritis, but it presents a classic Catch-22: Who wants to move when moving hurts? Countless arthritis sufferers have seen the relief the right workout program can offer. Follow these guidelines and you can be one of them:

◎ **Go low impact.** If you have arthritis, you must avoid high-impact exercise—anything that takes both feet off the ground at once, such as running (and all the sports that require it) and high-impact aerobics. For your aerobic workout, choose low-impact classes, walking, swimming, bicycling, and cardio exercise machines with padded tracks to complement your strength training, stretching, and balance routines.

◎ **Start slow.** Always warm up well before any workout session, moving each part of your body in an increasingly broad range of motion. If your joints are very stiff, take a warm shower or place a heating pad on the inflamed areas before you begin.

◎ **Time it right.** Exercise during the part of the day in which you have the least pain. For rheumatoid arthritis that may be later in the day, while early morning may be the best bet for osteoarthritis.

◎ **Listen to your joints as you exercise.** If you experience more pain than usual, stop for a while. If the pain continues, call it a day and try again tomorrow.

⊚ **Get wet.** If you have bad arthritis and can't tolerate weight-bearing exercise, put the buoyancy of water to work by exercising in a swimming pool. You'll get the same cardiovascular benefits without joint strain and improve your strength and balance all the while. Many health clubs and community pools offer aqua aerobics classes where you can learn how to exercise safely and without pain. While not as effective at building bones as weight-bearing exercise, water workouts can result in modest increases in bone mass as well as offer the many benefits of exercise.

NEW EXERCISE RULE #4:

PERSONALIZE YOUR EXERCISE PLAN

The AgeLess workouts that follow let you choose your intensity level, type of activities, and session length. Why is personal choice so important to successful exercise? Because the best exercise for you is the one you enjoy enough to continue. Of all the people who are prescribed fitness programs by their physicians, approximately half drop out within 6

America's Favorite Activities

Surveys of Americans' favorite forms of exercise find that low-impact activities get top marks. The activities we regularly engage in as a population include:

Walking (44%)
Gardening or yard work (29%)
Stretching (26%)
Bicycling (15%)
Strength training (14%)
Stair climbing (11%)
Jogging or running (9%)
Aerobics (7%)
Swimming (7%)

If you prefer a kinder, gentler workout, you have plenty of company, and you can easily maximize your longevity with your favorite exercises by following the AgeLess workouts.

months. In fact, at any given time, at least as many Americans are abandoning their exercise programs as starting them. That's why I developed a program that addresses one of the most common excuses: "I don't have time to exercise." For those who are more enthusiastic, I have the Basic AgeLess Workout that covers all the bases for aging less and the Ultimate AgeLess plan for fitness buffs.

In the aging equation, exercise is the most important variable. Staying active can protect you against the diseases of aging, guard your independence, and keep your brain working well, all while preserving the pleasures of youth—a fit body, good mood, sound sleep, satisfying sex, and the energy to live life to the fullest. Your body was built to move. To exercise your right to a long life, follow this divine plan every day and you may find yourself salsa dancing at your 100th birthday bash.

The I-Don't-Have-Time-to-Exercise Workout

Which of these is your excuse? "Too busy." "I don't have the energy." "I hate working out." If you and exercise are like oil and water, this is the plan for you. Designed in short bouts, these workouts slip easily into your schedule and boost your energy throughout the day. You don't even have to change your clothes—so exchange your excuses for a can-do, AgeLess exercise habit.

Aerobic
Three 10-minute breaks a day

- Park the car a little farther from work, shopping, or other locations and walk briskly to your destination.
- If you don't have to drive, leave the car at home and walk.
- Take the stairs instead of the elevator.
- Take a break from work with a fast walk around the floor or the block.
- Have lunch a little farther away from the office or house than usual and walk. Invite a colleague or friend to join you.
- Take the dog or a child for a walk.
- Do some housework or gardening.

AgeLess Tip: Keep a daily log in a small notebook or your handheld organizer to make sure you get your 30 minutes a day.

Strength Training
One 5-minute break a day

Pick up your hand weights or resistance bands and work four of your eight major muscle groups (see page 91). Tomorrow, tackle the other four.

AgeLess Tips: Keep a set of weights or bands at work for quick strength-training breaks. They don't take up much room and can even slide into a rack for easy storage and use. Welcome yourself home with 5 minutes of strength training in front of the television.

Flexibility and Balance
One 5-minute break a day

Take time to do some stretching and practice balance poses (see page 98). Great times to try to include:

- First thing in the morning
- Midafternoon slump at your desk
- Waiting for the pasta water to boil
- On your way to bed

AgeLess Tip: Play some soft, slow music while you stretch to help you relax.

The Basic AgeLess Workout

If you're ready to embrace exercise as your long-life elixir, the Basic AgeLess Workout is for you. Time-efficient and flexible, this is a template for fitness you can stick with for life.

45- to 55-minute session all or most days

Warm Up	Aerobics	Strength Training	Cool Down/Stretch
5 minutes	*30 minutes*	*10 minutes, twice a week*	*10 minutes*
Increase circulation and raise muscle temperature with large movements (arm and leg swings, knee lifts, walking or marching in place) and easy stretches.	Choose your favorite aerobic activity in your preferred exertion level from the list on page 84.	Using weight machines, free weights, or resistance bands, complete one set for each of the eight major muscle groups (see the exercises on page 91).	Walk or march until your heart rate returns to the resting level, then finish with flexibility and balance exercises (see page 98).

Exercise Made Easy

When asked why they don't work out regularly, most Americans have answers in common. Eliminate these exercise barriers with enabling solutions.

Exercise Obstacle	Exercise Enabler
Not enough time	Schedule small bouts throughout the day.
Lack of support from friends, family, and colleagues	Enlist a workout buddy and make regular exercise dates.
	Ask your partner for help with the kids or household tasks during your workout time.
	Make active recreation a family affair (try walking or bicycling together).
	Find a lunchtime walking buddy at work.
	Discuss business with the boss, fellow employees, or your staff while walking.
Marriage or significant relationship	Remember that you both deserve a longer healthspan in which to enjoy each other's company. Negotiate a workout schedule, either solo or à deux, that works for both of you.
Bad weather	Join a gym or buy a piece of cardio equipment and some handheld weights to do your workout at home.
	Walk the mall, climb the stairs at work, or head to an exercise studio where you can pay by the class.
Dislike pain and suffering	Take it easy on yourself! You don't have to suffer pain to enjoy the gains of exercise. Start with the I-Don't-Have-Time-to-Exercise Workout (see page 106).
Routine has been disrupted	Use 5- to 10-minute bouts to keep moving at least 30 minutes per day while you investigate your new options and settle on a revised routine that works for you.
No facilities or equipment	Walk! All you need is outdoor space or an indoor mall or stairs in bad weather. Back at home, finish with strength exercises (purchase one set of handheld weights or a resistance band) and a stretching routine.
Excess weight or disability	Exercise is critical to your quality of life now and to your AgeLess future. Consult your doctor about specific guidelines for safe activity, then use the information in this chapter to design your exercise program within your efficacy zone. Build up slowly and chart your progress.

The AgeLess Ultimate Workout

Designed to deliver greater challenge and rewards, this plan is suitable for people trying to maximize the benefits of exercise, maintain weight loss, achieve a highly toned physique—or with some extra time to invest in a longer, stronger life.

One 1- to 1½-hour session all or most days

Warmup	Aerobics	Strength Training	Cool Down/Stretch
5 minutes	*45 minutes*	*30 minutes, alternate days only*	*10 minutes*
Spur circulation and raise muscle temperature with large movements (arm and leg swings, knee lifts, walking or marching in place) and easy stretches.	Choose your favorite aerobic activity in your preferred exertion level from the list on page 84. Choose more vigorous activities for maximum conditioning benefits.	Using weight machines, free weights, or resistance bands, complete 1–3 sets for each of the eight major muscle groups (see the exercises on page 91).	Walk or march until your heart rate returns to the resting level, then finish with flexibility and balance exercises (see page 98)

HAVE AN AGELESS DAY

Exercise

Remember that you don't have to do all your daily exercise at the same time. Here's a sample day of cumulative exercise bouts that add up to an easy AgeLess workout without slowing you down.

- **8:30 A.M.** Park several blocks away from work or Starbucks and walk in briskly.
- **10:30 A.M.** Take the stairs at work or the shopping mall.
- **12:30 P.M.** Choose a lunch spot far enough away to give you an opportunity to stretch your legs or take a quick turn around the office, including stairs if you've got them.
- **3:00 P.M.** Afternoon slump calls for a quick stretching session. Adapt your exercises to your environment.
- **6:00 P.M.** Break out your handheld weights for some strength exercises before dinner.
- **9:00 P.M.** Start your sleeptime relaxation sequence with some yoga or tai chi movements.

YOUR AGELESS AGENDA
Exercise

Check off each item as you achieve it:

☐ Choose your personalized plan

☐ Cover the three exercise elements

1. Aerobic exercise: 30 minutes most or all days of the week
2. Strength training: Eight major muscle groups 10 to 20 minutes, 2 to 3 times a week
3. Flexibility and balance training: 5 to 10 minutes every day

☐ Use safety precautions and get expert instruction on proper form for lifting weights and using exercise machines

CHAPTER 4

WEIGHT

OLD WEIGHT RULE	NEW WEIGHT RULE
Thin is in.	**#1.** A few extra pounds could save your life.
Diet away those few extra pounds as many times as you need to.	**#2.** Unless you are seriously overweight or suffering from a weight-related disease, don't diet.
Watch the scale.	**#3.** Watch your waistline.
Believe the latest fad-diet promises.	**#4.** If you do need to lose weight, do it wisely.
Count calories to lose weight.	**#5.** Exercise for permanent weight loss.

I WAS SOUND ASLEEP when the phone rang. It was my mother, calling in the middle of the night from one of the world's leading health spas. She was on a 900-calorie-a-day diet, she said, and she was sleepless and miserable. After rubbing my eyes for a minute or two, I asked Mom why she was starving herself at a resort known for its good cuisine. She replied that the spa's staff told her that she needed to lose weight.

Weight is a torturous subject. Most of us want to reject the hard truth that between your thirties and your sixties or so, your body is programmed to gain weight as your metabolism slows. Even so, the ultra-lean figure has become a symbol of health and fitness.

Despite this widespread misconception that thinner is healthier, new research has shown that the thinnest people don't necessarily live longest or have the best health when they reach old age. And, as you can probably guess, neither do the heaviest. The ones who enjoy the greatest longevity are people in the middle of the weight range. Those rail-like figures in the fashion magazines rate low in weight longevity quotient. I don't know if you can be too rich, but you can indeed be too thin, especially as you age.

Don't get me wrong. Obesity—defined as having a body mass index, or BMI, of 30 and above—is a serious health problem in this country and around the world. It must be prevented and treated, and I'll discuss healthy weight loss later in this chapter. Still, unless you're obese or seriously overweight (a BMI of 27 to 29.9) or have a disease or risk profile that can be aggravated by extra body fat, you are more likely to undermine than improve your health by dieting. In fact, later in life, a little padding can protect against malnutrition and potentially disabling falls.

Let's get back to Mom, whom we've left sleepless and hungry at the health spa. Nineteen years ago, at age 72, my pleasantly plump mother definitely didn't need the draconian 900-calorie diet that the overzealous spa staff put her on. She didn't have diabetes, high blood pressure, arthritis, heart disease, or any other condition that would benefit from weight loss. Such a restrictive diet would be extreme for anyone. In a woman my mother's age, it could cause serious health problems. I advised Mom to enjoy her remaining vacation days savoring the delicious food the spa was renowned for.

In this chapter, I'll help you determine the weight that's best for you. With the information and tools in this chapter, you can stop agonizing about your weight and start adjusting your attitude toward an AgeLess relationship with body image and food.

WHAT'S YOUR LONGEVITY QUOTIENT?

Weight

Calculate your weight longevity quotient to determine where you stand in relation to the New Rules in this chapter. Before you start, there are three things you need to do.

1. Calculate your body mass index (BMI), a measure that relates weight to height, with the chart on pages 114 and 115 or the formula on the opposite page.

BMI: _____

2. Take a tape measure and measure your waistline just above the navel. Make sure the tape is level and snug but not tight or compressing the skin.

Waist circumference: _____ inches

Calculate Your Body Mass Index

You can also calculate your precise BMI with the following formula:

$$\text{BMI} = \frac{\text{weight (pounds)}}{\text{height (inches)}^2} \times 704.5 = \underline{\hspace{2cm}}$$

For example, I'm 6 feet (72 inches) tall and weigh 174 pounds. My BMI works out as follows:

$$\frac{174}{72^2\ (5,184)} \times 704.5 = 23.6$$

3. Check off all of the weight-related risk conditions that apply to you in the following list.

☐ Serious heart disease: previous heart attack, angina, coronary artery bypass surgery, angioplasty, or heart failure

☐ Other serious blood vessel diseases including stroke, aneurysm, or peripheral vascular disease

☐ High blood pressure ($\geq$ 140/90 millimeters of mercury)

☐ High blood cholesterol (total cholesterol $\geq$ 240 milligrams per deciliter or LDL $\geq$ 160 mg/dl) or high triglycerides ($\geq$ 150 mg/dl)

☐ Diabetes or prediabetic (high fasting blood sugar $\geq$ 110 milligrams)

☐ Smoke cigarettes or daily secondhand smoke exposure

☐ Sleep apnea (see chapter 5)

☐ Severe arthritis

☐ Gallbladder disease, including gallstones

☐ Sedentary lifestyle

Total number of weight-related risk factors: _____

Calculate Your Weight LQ

Now you're ready to translate your vital statistics into your weight LQ. Start by locating your BMI in the chart on page 116 and reading across for your raw score. Next, make adjustments for your exercise habits, age, waistline, and weight-related risk factors. Total the points for your final longevity quotient for weight.

(continued on page 116)

Calculate Your Body Mass Index

To find your body mass index (BMI), locate your height in the left column. Move across the chart (to the right) until you hit your approximate weight. Then follow that column down to the corresponding BMI number at the bottom of the chart.

Height	Weight (lb)						
4'10"	91	96	100	105	110	115	119
4'11"	94	99	104	109	114	119	124
5'0"	97	102	107	112	118	123	128
5'1"	100	106	111	116	122	127	132
5'2"	104	109	115	120	126	131	136
5'3"	107	113	118	124	130	135	141
5'4"	110	116	122	128	134	140	145
5'5"	114	120	126	132	138	144	150
5'6"	118	124	130	136	142	148	155
5'7"	121	127	134	140	146	153	159
5'8"	125	131	138	144	151	158	164
5'9"	128	135	142	149	155	162	169
5'10"	132	139	146	153	160	167	174
5'11"	136	143	150	157	165	172	179
6'0"	140	147	154	162	169	177	184
6'1"	144	151	159	166	174	182	189
6'2"	148	155	163	171	179	186	194
6'3"	152	160	168	176	184	192	200
6'4"	156	164	172	180	189	197	205
6'5"	160	168	176	185	193	202	210
6'6"	164	172	181	190	198	207	216
BMI	19	20	21	22	23	24	25

Height	Weight (lb)						
4'10"	124	129	134	138	143	148	153
4'11"	128	133	138	143	148	153	158
5'0"	133	138	143	148	153	158	163
5'1"	137	143	148	153	158	164	169
5'2"	142	147	153	158	164	169	174
5'3"	146	152	158	163	169	175	180
5'4"	151	157	163	169	174	180	186
5'5"	156	162	168	174	180	186	192
5'6"	161	167	173	179	186	192	198
5'7"	166	172	178	185	191	197	204
5'8"	171	177	184	190	197	203	210
5'9"	176	182	189	196	203	209	216
5'10"	181	188	195	202	208	215	222
5'11"	186	193	200	208	215	222	229
6'0"	191	199	206	213	221	228	235
6'1"	197	204	212	219	227	235	242
6'2"	202	210	218	225	233	241	249
6'3"	208	216	224	232	240	248	256
6'4"	213	221	230	238	246	254	263
6'5"	218	227	235	244	252	261	269
6'6"	224	233	241	250	259	267	276
BMI	26	27	28	29	30	31	32

WHAT'S YOUR LONGEVITY QUOTIENT?—(CONT.)

BMI	Raw LQ Score
Below 25	**100**
25–26.9	**90**
27–29.9	**70**
30–34.9	**50**
35 and above	**20**
Your Raw Score	_____

Add

10 points for regular exercise   _____

Add

10 points if you're age 55 or above   _____

Subtract

20 points if your waist is 40 inches or more (men)   (_____)
or 35 inches or more (women)

Subtract

20 points if your BMI is 25 or higher and you have two   (_____)
or more weight-related risk factors

Your Weight Longevity Quotient

(Cannot be over 100 or less than 0.)   _____

Here's how to interpret your LQ score for weight:

Total LQ Score	The Dean's Diagnosis
100	Congratulations! You're in the fit zone. Keep an eye on your waistline and exercise regularly. You can skip to the next chapter—unless you have the crazy idea that you can stand to lose a few pounds; in which case, read on.
90	You're technically overweight, but forget those hollow-faced waifs looking out from the magazine spreads. Losing weight won't make a big difference in your health and longevity, and dieting could diminish it. Ignore anyone who points out the extra pounds and just enjoy yourself—but don't gain any weight! And if you're set on shaping up, start exercising more.

80   You should shed a few pounds. If the word "spotty" best describes your exercise routine, start a daily program using the guidelines in this chapter. "Sensible" is your watchword. No fad diets and no diet pills, please!

70   It's time to get serious. You need to lose weight. Follow the weight-loss advice in this chapter and consult your doctor about other preventive measures.*

60 or less   Your longevity quotient is in jeopardy. Weight loss and exercise are your absolute top priorities. Follow the weight-loss advice in this chapter and consult your doctor about other preventive measures.*

*Screen for cholesterol, diabetes, and high blood pressure and treat if necessary.

Overweight Defined

Health experts divide body weight, as measured by BMI, into three categories: fit, overweight, and obese. According to the National Institutes of Health, your weight category by BMI is as follows:

Weight Category	BMI
Fit	Below 25
Overweight	25–29.9
Obese	30 and above

Fifty-five percent of Americans—about 97 million—are considered overweight or obese by this measure. I feel, however, that those between 25 and 26.9 should be considered borderline at most. Many people in this range are not, by any other measure, seriously overweight, and it's not until you get past 27 that you begin to see weight-related health problems. Most people in the borderline range will not serve their healthspans best by dieting.

Weight and Age

Most adults will see the number on the scale move up or down with different life stages. The fattening up in middle age and the slimming down or even wasting away in later years, to name two common fluctuations, are the natural result of many physiological changes that take place in our bodies over the course of our lifetimes. The good news is that, while they're normal, most of these changes can be slowed or min-imized by AgeLess habits. Here's what happens.

Your metabolic rate, or the speed at which you burn calories, slows down throughout middle age. This is, at least in part, a factor in the "middle-age spread" that so many of us dread in our thirties and forties. If you want to keep your weight gain to a minimum (about 2 pounds a decade is considered normal), watching what you eat is important, but don't diet unless your LQ indicates that you should. Your best bet for combating middle-age spread is exercise. Then, in your sixties, seventies, or eighties, the upward trend in weight starts to turn around—but this is not necessarily good news. Many individuals experience an ironic shift from trying to eat less to worrying about not eating enough. Nutritional status is a serious concern as appetites diminish and other physical changes make it harder for many older people to get adequate nutrition.

As you age, your tastebuds and smell receptors become less efficient, dulling the pleasure of food and diminishing the desire to eat. At this stage of life, there's a good chance that your social networks may also start to unravel, making it less likely that you will sit down and enjoy a good

What to Expect When . . .

Here are some of the weight-related signposts you might encounter as time goes by.

- ⑥ **Twenties:** These are your "reference weight" years. Weight gain from here on in is associated with increased risk of type 2 diabetes.
- ⑥ **Thirties:** Age-related weight gain begins, an accumulation of fat that stems from reduced physical activity and loss of muscle mass. This problem is mostly behavioral—and you can prevent it with New Rule #5.
- ⑥ **Forties:** Middle-age weight gain continues unless combated with diet and exercise.
- ⑥ **Fifties:** Peak weight years for most. After about age 55, keeping weight up can become a concern.
- ⑥ **Sixties:** Average BMI starts to decline with health problems that inter-fere with appetite, cooking, or both, and waning social support.
- ⑥ **Seventies and eighties:** Obesity rates decline, possibly because many obese individuals have already died. Adequate nutrition becomes critical to protect against illness and to keep weight at life-sustaining levels.

meal on a regular basis. Arthritis or other physical conditions can make grocery shopping and cooking an arduous chore. And, though this may be hard to imagine now if chewing and swallowing are two of your best-developed skills, medical and dental conditions can make eating difficult.

As a result of all these changes, many older people start eating less than they need. Even in healthy older folks, this can result in dangerously inadequate intake of protein, vitamins, and minerals. For someone frail, such a shortfall can be fatal, especially during illness or following an injury. As noted in chapter 2, your risk of falling and breaking bones rises as the years go by. And this is where those few extra pounds come in handy: Some natural cushioning can make the difference between a bruise and a hip fracture.

The importance of adequate body weight to a healthy old age is borne out by the data. In a study of 7,000 individuals over age 70, people who weighed in the lowest 10 percent spent more time in hospitals and died younger than those in the middle of the weight range. This differential wasn't caused by sickness in the underweight group; those with cancer, heart disease, and diabetes were screened out (of course, this probably excluded people in the high weight range as well). Among healthy participants, each additional increment of weight actually increased survival rates.

A 20-year study of Americans ages 55 to 74 found the lowest mortality rates among people with BMIs from 25 to 30, which is overweight according to federal standards but may be just right for seniors.

NEW WEIGHT RULE #1:
A FEW EXTRA POUNDS COULD SAVE YOUR LIFE

The great novelist and social commentator, Tom Wolfe, captured our national obsession with thinness in his best-selling novel *The Bonfire of the Vanities*. His depiction of emaciated socialites on New York's Upper East Side sums up how we've come to equate the look of hunger with status, sexuality, and achievement. For most of the past four decades, fashion magazines have exclusively featured gaunt, bony models. A weight gain of even a few pounds might jeopardize an actress's Hollywood career. Thin is in, and fat is frowned upon. But for all our skinny dreams, the majority of Americans are officially overweight and losing their battles with the bulge, engaged in a destructive cycle of yo-yo dieting and diminishing self-esteem that can be very detrimental to their healthspans.

Take the Long View

Most people don't think beyond the next few months when considering weight-related matters—but a long view of what happens to your weight as you age is the best way to optimize healthspan, through middle-age spread and the surprising slim-down you're likely to see in later years. To utilize the Longevity Quotient Plan for weight, forget the quick fixes pushed down your throat by the diet industry and focus only on changes that you can comfortably make for life.

Adding to the media message that thinner is more attractive is the popular belief that a low calorie diet tips the odds in favor of a longer life. If you enjoy eating, you'll be happy to know that there's no scientific evidence that this is true for human beings.

The research on calorie restriction and longevity started when scientists who were working with lab rats and mice found that when the little critters were fed low-calorie diets, they lived longer. Not only did the hungry rodents look and act younger, they developed fewer tumors and other diseases than animals that ate freely. My friend Dr. Roy Walford, one of the great pioneers in aging research, has restricted the calories and maximized the nutrients consumed by adult mice and seen them live significantly longer than mice who ate regular rations.

Some scientists would like to extrapolate these experimental animal results to human beings. Dr. Walford, for instance, has written the "125-Year" diet plan with a rock-bottom calorie count that he proposes could increase human lifespans to a century and a quarter. Is he right?

Dr. Walford's diet might do the trick for the rodent residents of his lab, but there's no evidence that the life-extending effects of near-starvation apply to people. Clearly, food deprivation during famine or war has shortened, rather than lengthened, human lifespan. Granted, such tragedies are not controlled scientific studies, but the problem is that we don't have any of those. No sizable group of people has ever followed Dr. Walford's low-calorie, highly supplemented nutrient regimen long enough to measure its effect on longevity. Chances are good that there never will be such a group of volunteers, since the austere calorie allowance would probably prohibit you from ever eating another full meal again, and there's no sign that any animal with free access to food will willingly live with hunger over the long term. Even if we were to develop such iron wills, the result may well be a shorter, not longer, healthspan. The reason for this reprieve is a reassuring phenomenon known as the "J curve."

Living in the Middle of the J Curve

Life insurance companies have always been interested in predicting how long we'll live, and over the years their actuaries have compiled vast databases of the weights, heights, and lifespans of millions of individuals. This rich repository of information together with the results of clinical research studies reveal a J-curve relationship between weight and mortality—that is, the highest mortality rates are found in people with the lowest and highest BMIs. The longest-lived group is in the middle weight categories.

Where exactly is the sweet spot on the J curve that promises the longest life? A 14-year study of more than 1 million Americans found the

Comparing the J and U Curves

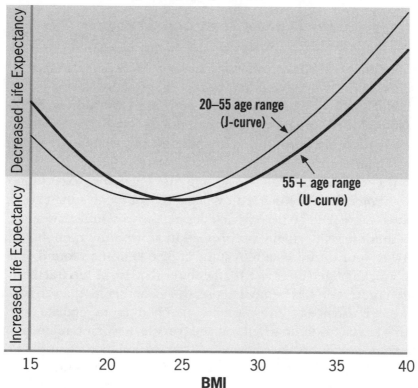

greatest life expectancy at BMIs of 22 to 28 overall. A 1999 study that tracked more than 1 million adults over 14 years pinpointed the weight range with the lowest mortality rates for women and men. Here's where the statistics place the sweet spot for different population groups.

Population Group	BMI	Population Group	BMI
White women	18.5–28.0	African-American women	18.5–30.0
White men	20.5–28.0	African-American men	22.0–25.0

Though the federal government considers you overweight at a BMI of 25 or above, your body doesn't seem to mind—unless you are at risk for diseases like diabetes and high blood pressure, where those extra pounds make the difference between health and disease.

With aging, the J-shaped curve changes shape. The lopsided J, which favors being underweight more than overweight, turns into a U. In later years, the perils of being underweight catch up with the life-expectancy costs of being overweight. Being obese at any age is dangerous.

The Pluses of Those Last 10 Pounds

Fat is nothing more or less than our body's storage bin, and nature provided these fuel reserves for a reason—a few reasons, in fact.

First, you may need to draw on your energy stores if you get sick or hurt. Healing from illness or injury requires extra calories, but many people lose their appetite under such duress, especially in older age. The deficit can literally kill you if you don't carry any spare weight to cover the difference.

A few extra pounds can also act as a shock absorber to cushion your bones if you fall. With hip fractures being one of the deadliest accidents around—more than 20 percent of older people who suffer a hip fracture die within the year—some soft protection around the hipbone can be pivotal to your future health. A study of 35,000 women found that the more weight gained after age 18, the lower the risk of hip fracture. The greatest protection was found in those who gained more than 25 pounds.

Women also need a baseline amount of body fat to regulate estrogen levels, a key factor in how well you age. Very lean women often lack the body fat needed for proper hormonal balance and may experience thinning bones, dry skin, and other evidence of accelerated aging as a result of low estrogen levels.

NEW WEIGHT RULE #2:

UNLESS YOU ARE SERIOUSLY OVERWEIGHT OR SUFFERING FROM A WEIGHT-RELATED DISEASE, DON'T DIET

Not only can those spare pounds protect your health, but trying to peel them off may lower your chances of successful aging. Many people have died in the drive to diet. From the risks of nutritional imbalance to dangerous medications, dieting can be dangerous—and the effort is rarely successful in the long term.

One study found that a weight loss of more than 4.5 percent of body weight (not disease-related) increased women's risk of death within the next 6 years by *four times over*. That's quite a blow to longevity for, say, a 150-pound person taking off a little less than 7 pounds. Nonetheless, companies that push diet plans and products thrive on our anxiety about the weight game, and business is booming. Americans spend billions of dollars on diet products each year, including numerous pills and programs with no scientific basis at all. While government agencies such as the FDA try to keep a watch on the weight-watching industry, they are woefully understaffed and can only stop a few of the most fraudulent scams.

Most Diets Don't Work

There aren't many laws against spreading misinformation through books, and when it comes to diet books, it's a case of "buyer beware." Many of the most popular diet books, especially the bestsellers, rely on something-for-nothing gimmicks and utterly fail to provide the nutrition you need for optimal longevity. (Certainly, there are many responsible diet books available, but they rarely make it to the top of the bestsellers list.)

For instance, today's popular high-protein diets could lower your life

Everybody's Doing It

What's our national passion? Apparently, dieting. The most recent National Health and Nutrition Examination Survey (NHANES I) found that 53 percent of women and 30 percent of men had tried to lose weight in the previous year. No wonder the diet industry rakes in more than $30 billion a year!

expectancy by promoting heart disease, straining your kidneys, leaching calcium from bones, and depriving you of the antioxidants plentiful in the many forbidden or restricted fruits and vegetables. Some of the advice offered by diet books borders on the bizarre. One popular plan suggests that chocolate mousse is okay, but carrots are harmful! It looks as though chocolate does have health-promoting properties, as I mentioned in chapter 2, but I don't think "reducing aid" is one of them. If eating chocolate mousse could really lead to weight loss, I'd be several pounds lighter. As for carrots, they're packed with carotenoid compounds that may protect against many life-threatening diseases, and they make great snacks for longevity and health.

In 2001, the American Heart Association (AHA) published a review of high-protein, low-carbohydrate diets such as the Zone and Atkins. High-protein diets (those in which protein comprises 30 percent or more of calories) got very low marks. The AHA criticized these plans on numerous points that directly affect healthspan: promoting high levels of saturated fat; restricting certain fruits and vegetables, which contain the very nutrients you need for maximum health; and providing inadequate fiber. Any success claimed by these diets results from the basic fact that any plan limiting calories will produce weight loss. The AHA concluded that people who follow high-protein programs are at risk for inadequate micronutrient intake and heart, liver, kidney, and bone diseases and disorders. Similar warnings apply to any number of fad diets.

The deprivation of dieting can also dull your quality of life. Constant food obsession, calorie counting, anguish over every bite swallowed and each step onto the scale, and self-recrimination for the very smallest "failure" are common characteristics of the dieter's mentality. While smart food choices are an important element of successful aging, letting food anxiety control you can seriously sap your happiness and the daily joy that makes life worth living.

And for all the effort, what's the usual end result? Of those dieters who manage to lose a significant amount—10 percent of total body weight or more—a staggering 80 percent put back on every pound—and often more—which is as hard on your body as it is on your spirit and self-esteem. Picture this scenario: You just started your diet plan, you're going to the gym every day, and your two best friends are partnering on the project. Within several weeks you've lost 15 pounds, and your wife is crazy about your new svelte figure. You're a slim success!

Flash ahead 6 months. Your schedule gets too busy for you to keep up your gym routine, the repetitive packaged meals are long beyond boring, your two best friends have fallen off the wagon, and your wife takes the lost weight for granted and slacks off on the praise. Are you going to maintain your hard-won weight loss—or start slipping up as the thrill of victory fades and you face the many temptations of daily life?

Ample evidence shows that yo-yo dieting is the rule in the weight-loss game, and that the roller-coaster ride harms health and makes losing weight more difficult in the future. How high a price are you willing to pay for a few pounds that you'll probably put on again anyway?

Warning: Diet Pills Can Be Hazardous to Your Health

While fad or restrictive diets alone can be dangerous, the medications that many people take in the quest for thinness can seriously compound the problem. Several diet drugs have been associated with health risks, from digestive disorders to heart damage and sudden death.

Still fresh in our memories is the tragedy of fen-phen, a combination of fenfluramine and phentermine that caused many unwitting dieters to experience heart valve damage from the drug. These drugs (fen-phen and Redux) are also associated with a deadly disease called primary pulmonary hypertension. By 1997, when fen-phen was recalled, some 10 million prescriptions had been written. The terrible toll of this mistake may continue to haunt those who have taken the drugs for years to come.

For individuals whose BMI is 30 or more, or 27-plus with the weight-related risk factors or diseases described in this chapter, some drugs are appropriate to aid dieting. Sibutramine (Meridia), which works by blocking reuptake of the neurotransmitter serotonin to enhance feelings of satisfaction, is one such drug. Some people experience a small rise in blood pressure as a side effect. Another is the diet drug orlistat (Xenical), which blocks an enzyme required to absorb ingested fat. The good news is that since it reduces fat absorption, it lowers caloric intake and cholesterol levels. But guess where all that undigested fat goes? In the drug's first major trial, 38 percent of participants experienced diarrhea, bloating, and flatulence.

Prescription diet drugs should only be taken in the lowest possible doses, under a doctor's direct care, and in the context of a healthy diet and exercise program designed to modify your lifestyle. If your personal profile doesn't call for diet drugs, you must avoid them to maximize your healthspan.

Over-the-counter remedies carry their own risks. Ephedra, an herb found in many "natural" diet aids, is a powerful stimulant to the central nervous system that can cause seizures, high blood pressure, increased heart rate and heart palpitations, and stroke. Several deaths have been attributed to ephedra—10 in one 21-month period. Phenyl-propanolamine (PPA, an ingredient in the supplement Lipokinetix and many cold remedies) is another nonprescription diet aid associated with hemorrhagic stroke, the most devastating kind. The FDA has advised that PPA be taken off the market, but products containing the substance still circulate through Web sites and other purveyors hoping to snag wishful thinkers who believe that a pill can "mimic exercise" in the human body.

A 2001 study reported in the *Journal of the American Medical Association* (*JAMA*) set out to determine how many people were taking non-prescription diet aids, including PPA and ephedra. A full 7 percent of those surveyed reported use of nonprescription diet drugs over the 2-year study period, which is quite a large segment of the general population. Among them were 29 percent of young obese women. But here's the real surprise: 8 percent of normal-weight women took PPA and ephedra, needlessly spending money and putting their health at risk for no apparent reason.

NEW WEIGHT RULE #3:

WATCH YOUR WAISTLINE

As you age, you're likely to see a southward slide of any extra fat. Starting in your thirties, you may lose fat in your arms and upper body only to add bulges to your hips, thighs, and waist—and in this redistribution, location matters. Evidence shows that too much abdominal fat is probably a bigger alarm for increased risk of cardiovascular disease, high blood pressure, and diabetes than a high BMI—so much so that the New Rule is to pay more attention to your waistline than the scale when deciding whether or not to diet.

To protect your health and vitality, you want to watch carefully for development of the "apple" shape created by abdominal fat—a sign that the inevitable downward slide has crossed the line into a health hazard—whether manifested as one of those big beer bellies you might bump into at an NFL game or a more subtly thickened midriff. Researchers aren't yet sure why large waistlines are such a health hazard, but it's clear that

Your Abdominal Shape: Apple versus Pear

Compare your silhouette to these two shapes. It's best for your healthspan to avoid the acquired apple profile. If you were born to look like a pear, don't worry.

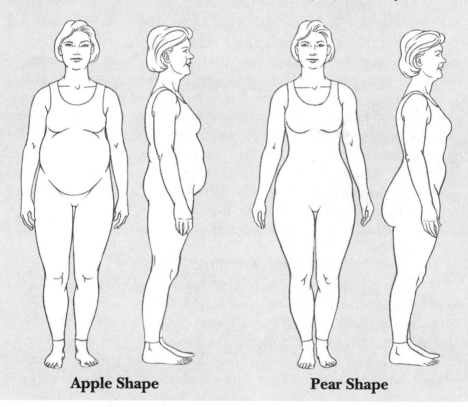

Apple Shape   **Pear Shape**

extra weight is more dangerous when it's located around your middle. Far better for your health is to be shaped like a pear, as exemplified in the paintings of Rubens and Renoir and the illustrations above. A few spare pounds on the hips and thighs, an inborn rather than acquired condition, appear to do little harm to your health.

Abdominal fat is such an important indicator that the National Institutes of Health now recommends measuring your waistline to judge whether you need to lose weight. You should have already done this in assessing your longevity quotient for weight. Girths of 35 inches or above for women and 40 inches or above for men indicate excessive abdominal fat. If you fall into this danger zone, read on. New Rules #4 and #5 will tell you what to do.

NEW WEIGHT RULE #4:

IF YOU DO NEED TO LOSE WEIGHT, DO IT WISELY

While a few extra pounds can be beneficial, once your weight moves past the middle of the J or U curves into the range of serious overweight and obesity, your risk of a shorter healthspan increases dramatically. Though many in the low overweight range (BMI of 25 to 26.9) don't need to sweat the extra pounds, plenty of people do have weight to lose. If you have a predisposition to or early signs of high blood pressure, diabetes, sleep apnea, gallbladder or cardiovascular disease, a few less pounds could make the difference in developing these conditions. For people with arthritis, a little less weight on those joints could reduce your pain. A study of individuals who were prediabetic showed that losing a few pounds together with extra exercise and fiber could prevent 58 percent of them from developing diabetes. If your weight LQ is 80 or less, talk to your doctor about the advisability of weight loss.

Overweight: America's Epidemic

Despite all our diets and rows of low-fat foods on supermarket shelves, Americans continue to gain weight, moving toward the treacherous upward slope of the J curve. Since 1980, adult obesity rates have doubled. In 2001, the U.S. Surgeon General deemed the situation so serious that he issued an official call to action, warning that rising rates of obesity and overweight could reverse advances we've made in heart disease, cancer, and other chronic health problems during recent decades. Being overweight or obesity account for an estimated 300,000 deaths a year, close on the heels of cigarette smoking (400,000).

And 47 million American adults—more than one in five—are estimated to suffer from a disorder that the National Institutes of Health has recently dubbed "metabolic syndrome." Defined as a cluster of weight-related conditions, metabolic syndrome involves having three or more of the following interrelated conditions:

- Excess abdominal fat (beer belly)
- Elevated blood pressure
- Excess blood sugar levels
- High triglycerides (fats that circulate in the blood)
- Cholesterol imbalance (low HDL)

Reducing Can Reverse Disease

Topping the list of the deadly consequences of being seriously overweight or obesity is cardiovascular disease—our nation's number one killer. Obese individuals are *50 to 100 percent more likely* to develop cardiovascular disease than people in the fit range. Gaining weight raises the risk of a heart attack by 25 percent for 11 to 18 additional pounds and by a formidable 250 percent with a gain of 44 pounds. Risk for ischemic stroke (the most common type, in which a blood vessel to the brain ruptures) increases with BMI. A woman with a BMI over 27 is at 75 percent greater risk than one whose BMI is under 21, while risk is 137 percent higher at BMIs over 32. Too much extra weight can also drive up your blood pressure. Studies find that 22 extra pounds can increase blood pressure enough to raise your estimated risk for heart disease by 12 percent and for stroke by 24 percent. Cholesterol is another concern. Both higher body weight and excess abdominal fat are associated with increasing total and LDL cholesterol levels.

If you're a smoker, however, it's unwise to assess your heart disease risk strictly by body weight and the related risk factors. People who smoke tend to have lower BMIs but higher rates of heart disease than the nonsmoking population. Smoking is never a wise weight-management tool.

Many other diseases are associated with being significantly overweight. The risk of developing adult-onset (type 2) diabetes increases 25 percent with each additional BMI unit. A widening waistline is another risk factor for type 2 diabetes. Weight is also a risk factor for colon, breast, and endometrial cancers. The Nurses' Health Study found twice the risk for distal colon cancer among women with a BMI over 29 than

Smokers: Go Ahead and Kick the Habit

If you smoke, the single most significant step you can take to increase your healthspan is to stop. But many potential quitters worry about gaining weight, and with reason. About 80 percent of people who stop smoking do put on pounds—on average, about 5 to 7. This may make your clothes tight but is hardly a health concern anywhere near that of carcinogenic smoke.

If you're ready to quit smoking but are concerned about weight gain, I recommend that you monitor your calories and keep them at maintenance level during your cessation program. If your weight LQ indicates a need for weight loss, wait until well after you've kicked the habit to take on that challenge.

those with one under 21, and a large waist girth is associated with prevalence of colon polyps. In the 10 years after menopause, there's a direct link between obesity and breast cancer mortality. Fatty tissue, the primary source of estrogen in postmenopausal women, is a primary risk factor for breast cancer. And risk for endometrial cancer is three times higher for women with a BMI over 30 than for normal-weight women, and it also rises with adult weight gain.

Excess weight also puts pressure on your joints, which can cause or aggravate arthritis. As an example, one study estimated that the risk of developing osteoarthritis increases by 9 to 13 percent with every additional kilogram (2.2 pounds) of body weight. Women experience a stronger association between extra weight and knee arthritis than men do.

If you're overweight with two or more of the risk factors outlined in the Longevity Quotient quiz or if you're obese, you need to lose weight. Even modest weight loss can lower high blood pressure enough that you may no longer need to take hypertension medications. Weight loss can also bring down elevated blood sugar levels and reduce or eliminate your need for antidiabetic drugs. Important to much of the population is the power of weight loss in reducing bad (LDL) cholesterol and boosting good (HDL) cholesterol levels, which in turn can reduce your risk of heart disease, heart attacks, and stroke. If you have arthritis, particularly involving your hips, knees, or ankles, slimming down can ease the strain on these damaged joints. Excess body *fat* is also one of the "four Fs" that increase the risk of gallbladder disease, along with being *female*, previous *fertility* (giving birth), and having crossed your *fortieth* birthday. As you can see, weight is the only factor you can modify to prevent this condition.

Achieve Your AgeLess Weight

By now you understand that weight can work both ways. The Age-Less strategy is to stay trim for good health in your early and middle years and allow a few pounds to cushion you in your older age.

If you scored 100 on the weight LQ quiz, skip this section. Those who scored 90 should read on to find out about how to keep pounds from accumulating in the future. If your weight LQ rates 80 or lower, it's time to reduce. Fortunately, the days of drastic diet recommendations are pretty much past. Current evidence shows that small increments of weight loss may be your best bet for treating most medical conditions. Losing just 10 percent of body weight is the benchmark goal for improving health

Rate Your Weight-Loss Motivation

Answer each of the following questions to rate your weight-loss motivation. For questions 2 to 5, rate each item on a scale of 1 to 5, with 5 being the highest or most important.

1. Number of previous weight-loss attempts _____
2. Desire to improve health and longevity _____
3. Support from family, friends, and workplace _____
4. Willingness and ability to exercise _____
5. Time available for attention to diet and exercise _____
6. Length of honest commitment to keeping the weight off (0: haven't thought about it; 1: 6 months or less; 2: 6 months to 1 year; 3: 1 to 2 years; 4: more than 2 years; 5: for life) _____

To score, add up your points for questions 2 to 6. Subtract your points for question 1. Your total score _____

Your Score	Diet-Readiness Rating
20–25	Go for it! You're motivated for lasting success.
15–19	You could probably get started on a weight-loss program today, but you might want to think ahead to a month from now. Remind yourself of the importance of healthier eating habits and make sure you're in it for the long haul.
10–14	You know you *should* diet, but you're not that thrilled with the idea. Examine your resistance and make sure you really feel committed before you get started.
9 or less	Let's face it—you're not ready. Consider therapy or a support group to help you examine your "issues" about weight. It may be the most important AgeLess decision you'll ever make.

among those in the range of risk. Such moderate weight loss is so effective that more radical regimens are generally only recommended in extreme cases, after the initial weight loss has stabilized. In fact, evidence that losing more than 10 percent of body weight may reduce metabolic rate and help explain why it can be so difficult to maintain larger losses.

Before you embark on a weight-loss program, it's important to do a little planning. Here are three advance steps that will help you achieve your goal.

1. Assess your motivation. The question is, "Why diet?" When your answer penetrates beyond surface appearances and social pressures to encompass the deeper payoff of a healthy body weight, you're ready to go.

Initial Weight-Loss Goal

Pounds to lose (10 percent of your present body weight)   _____ pounds

Goal weight (present weight − pounds to lose)   _____ pounds

Number of weeks (pounds to lose ÷ 1 or 2 pounds per week)   _____ weeks

Goal date (start date + number of weeks)   _____

Your goal date is nothing more than a motivational aid. If your weight loss goes more slowly than you planned, don't panic or give up. Simply recalculate your goal date based on your actual weight-loss rate and continue with your program.

If your goal includes enjoying better health and energy today, preventing debilitating disease in the future, and maximizing your healthspan, you're prepared to take the plunge.

2. Set your goal. Your initial AgeLess goal is to lose 10 percent of your current body weight at the rate of 1 to 2 pounds per week. You can probably accomplish this safely over the course of about 6 months or less. Faster is not better for losing weight, and trying to accelerate the process will only stress your body; spur metabolic resistance, thereby slowing weight loss; and make it harder to stick to your plan. Use the chart above to set your initial weight-loss goal.

After meeting your initial weight-loss goal, recalculate your BMI and measure your waist. Check your new numbers against the LQ weight quiz on page 112.

- If your score is now 90 or above, congratulate yourself and move on to a maintenance plan.
- If your updated weight LQ is 80 or below, you still have some weight to lose, but don't rush it! Instead, take 6 months on a maintenance plan to allow your weight to stabilize while your body and mind adjust to your new lifestyle. After 6 months of maintenance, repeat the goal-setting process and return to the weight-loss program. Repeat the full cycle as many times as necessary to bring your weight LQ up to 90.

3. Find the diet plan that works for you. While new diet plans seem to hit the stands every day, most of them are based on dramatic, unrealistic promises of rapid weight loss and lack the central element of success: scientific, evidence-based guidelines. In 1998, the National Institutes of Health finally filled the knowledge gap with a landmark analysis of published scientific research to set guidelines for how to achieve the most effective, lasting weight loss with the greatest health benefits.

This sophisticated synthesis of scientific knowledge was unprecedented. By categorizing research evidence, evaluating its significance and strength, and translating the results into concrete recommendations, the NIH initiative brought robust science to the pseudoscientific rhetoric that permeates the diet industry. And what does it all boil down to? Controlling calories and getting plenty of exercise.

A Calorie By Any Other Name

Let me reintroduce you to a simple but seemingly forgotten key to weight loss: the calorie. While many fad diets will try to fool you into thinking that the nature of a calorie varies from one food to another, this isn't true. A calorie is a calorie—a concise, constant scientific measure of the energy value of any given food. Excess energy from any source is stored in the body as fat, while an energy deficit causes fat to be burned. The only way to lose weight is to eat fewer calories than you

(continued on page 136)

AGELESS MYTH BUSTER
Calories Don't Count

MYTH

Some calories are more fattening than others.

FACT

A calorie is a calorie is a calorie. Every calorie supplies the same amount of energy to the body. The cause of most calorie confusion is that foods vary in their caloric *density*. Fat packs in 9 calories per gram, while protein and carbohydrates supply less than half as much energy by weight—4 calories per gram. Most foods are a mix of these nutrients, water, and undigested substances (fiber). So at the end of the day, consulting the calorie count and portion size on the package label is the best way to gauge the energy value of the food you eat.

Diets that claim to burn fat through special biochemical reactions (for instance, the Zone, which touts insulin control as its magic bullet) are nothing more than low-calorie diets in disguise.

Top 10 Tips for Permanent Weight Loss

At Carrie Wiatt's Diet Designs in Los Angeles, dieters from all walks of life discover an important truth: Weight loss should last for life. A nutritionist and author who frequently appears in the media to explain the science of losing weight safely and the art of eating well, Wiatt specializes in helping people make the lifetime commitment that eludes so many dieters. If you are overweight with risk factors or are obese, Wiatt's top 10 tips can significantly expand your healthspan.

1. **Have a plan.** You've heard the adage that people who fail to plan are planning to fail. When it comes to losing weight, a comprehensive plan that covers your menus, exercise, support networks, and progress assessments is key. Make sure that you choose a plan that works for you.

2. **Go slow.** The optimum rate for lasting weight loss is 1 to 2 pounds a week, which works out to a deficit of 500 to 1,000 calories a day. If you're over age 50, the deficit should be closer to 500 calories. To prevent frustration and stress, turn your attention away from the scale and concentrate on how you feel and how your clothes fit. Weigh yourself no more than once a week, and remember that occasional plateaus are normal even when you're adhering to your plan.

3. **Control your portions.** Weight loss is a matter of consuming fewer calories than you burn—and most Americans eat 1,000 calories more per day than they realize. Here's how to resize the eating blueprint in your mind.

   ✆ Take a day to measure everything you currently eat, from orange juice and cereal to your sandwich at lunch, the baked potato at dinner, snacks—everything. Use both quantitative measuring tools (cups and the scale) and visual ones (a regular, digital, or video camera).

   ✆ Take another day to measure and record your portions according to your new eating plan.

   ✆ Downsize your plates to create a healthier portion perception. Use a salad plate instead of a dinner plate, replace a tall tumbler with a juice glass, and skip super-size containers at the supermarket, restaurant, or take-out counter.

4. **Learn to navigate a restaurant menu.** One of the chief causes of our national portion problem is oversize servings at restaurants. Here's an easy rule of thumb: If you're eating out or getting takeout, cut your order in half. If half-size portions aren't available, share with a companion or ask to have the dish split in the kitchen and the other half packed to take home. Or ask your waiter about portion sizes or look at the plates of other diners.

5. **Count calories, not grams of fat.** It's your total energy intake that determines whether you burn, maintain, or store body fat, so you need to control your overall calorie count, not just cut back fat, in order to lose weight. Limit fat to 30 percent of total calories to leave room for important nutrients.

6. **Eat frequently.** Interval eating, or a regular schedule of small meals and snacks throughout the day, selected from your weight-loss meal plan, can help keep your blood sugar stable, prevent hunger, and support efficient digestion and fat burning.

7. **Spend your calories wisely.** Focus on fruits, vegetables, whole grains, legumes, low-fat dairy, and lean protein sources to get the nutritional mix that will keep you looking and feeling great while you lose weight.

8. **Journal your food every day.** Writing down exactly what and how much you eat keeps you accountable for your actions. A written record also helps you spot portion problems, eating triggers, and ways to improve your diet's balance.

9. **Exercise the other side of the energy equation.** Weight loss comes from burning more calories than you eat, and exercise is a critical part of the equation. Studies show that people who exercise regularly have the best success at losing weight and keeping it off.

10. **Seek support.** Losing weight can be a big job, but you don't have to do it alone. Working with a nutritionist, joining a program or group, and signing on to chat rooms and bulletin boards on the Internet are all wonderful support options. Be sure to stay in touch with your support network after the weight is lost. Maintenance is the hardest part!

For Wiatt's program for weight loss and maintenance, see her book *Portion Savvy: The 30-Day Smart Plan for Eating Well.* You can also find a diet matched to your personality style in her *Eating by Design: The Individualized Food Personality Type Nutrition Plan,* or stop by www.DietDesigns.com.

expend. Whether those calories come from carrots, chocolate, or chicken breast, if you take in at the end of the day less than the total you've burned up, you lose weight. That's all there is to it.

To help you out with the calorie connection, I tapped nutritionist and author Carrie Wiatt, who is nationally known for helping people re-size their portion pictures in their minds (see "Carrie Wiatt's Top 10 Tips for Permanent Weight Loss" on page 134). Carrie's book *Portion Savvy* revealed the secret she uses to keep some of Hollywood's top stars slim: balancing your energy equation through portion control. This is a scientifically sound way to lose weight, and it works.

Consult your doctor before beginning any weight-loss program. Medical supervision is particularly important if you are pregnant or have any major health condition.

NEW WEIGHT RULE #5:
EXERCISE FOR PERMANENT WEIGHT LOSS

I can't say it emphatically enough: The most important factor in your weight-loss success is exercise.

Managing Your Weight Naturally

In general, I don't endorse diet aids (other than prescription medications for certain individuals as I've described). There are many natural boosts available, however, to your weight-management efforts.

- **Fiber:** The fiber found in fruits, vegetables, whole grains, bran, and dried beans can help keep you feeling full and stabilize blood sugar levels. Fiber is a dieter's friend!
- **Water:** Even more vital to life than food, water is such a primal need that people frequently confuse thirst for hunger. Two quarts a day will flush away toxins and promote a feeling of fullness. Herbal teas and diet soft drinks can supplement your water regimen, but steer clear of sweetened sodas and juices, which can pack on the calories and pounds.
- **Self-care treatments:** A hot bath, massage, facial mask, foot soak, aromatherapy—from simple home remedies to special treats at the spa, any self-care routines that make you feel good can improve your mood, fuel your motivation, and keep you out of the kitchen.

Throughout adulthood, the rate at which most bodies burn energy—calories from food—starts to decline by about 2 percent per decade, and with this slowdown generally comes weight gain. If you feel as though you can't eat what you could 10 years ago without packing on pounds, you're probably right. Likewise, lower metabolic rate means that weight you put on in later years is particularly hard to take off. But buck up, midlifers! You have the power to stop this metabolic meltdown in its tracks. While middle-age spread was once seen as inevitable, more recent research pegs it to lack of exercise and resulting loss of muscle mass.

If you're looking to lose weight and keep it off for good, take some tips from the nation's most successful maintainers. The National Weight Control Registry tracks dieters who have lost at least 30 pounds and kept it off for a year or more. They report four habits in common, and the number one habit is regular exercise. Successful maintainers burned 2,700 calories per week—about an hour of moderate exercise a day. See chapter 3 for more about exercising to counter metabolic slowdown and maximize your LQ.

The other secrets to long-term weight-loss success uncovered by the National Weight Control Registry include following a low-fat, high-carbohydrate diet. As I've noted and contrary to some fad diet plan claims, piling on the protein doesn't make you slim. Of course, piling on anything is not a sound diet technique, and furthermore some carbohydrates are better than others. Chapter 2 provides an AgeLess Nutrition Pyramid to help you make AgeLess food choices in the context of your weight-loss plan.

AGELESS TIP

Plan Ahead

"Be prepared" is a good motto for any project, but it's especially important to plan ahead when making a lifestyle change. To prevent inertia and old habits from stopping you in your tracks, start your weight-loss program by sitting down and scheduling your first week of meals and exercise sessions. Keep the power of planning on your side by continuing to schedule menus and workouts at least a few days in advance until your AgeLess habits are in place.

HAVE AN AGELESS DAY
Weight

Here are some easy ways to follow the New Rules for weight today and every day.

- ⟲ **Greet** the day by affirming your commitment to improving your healthspan, the healthy part of lifespan.
- ⟲ **Eat** at least three evenly spaced meals that emphasize healthy foods.
- ⟲ **Meet** your daily exercise requirement.
- ⟲ **Sneak in** extra exercise anywhere you can—climbing the stairs, parking farther from a store, walking the dog, cleaning the house.
- ⟲ **Switch** pictures: Put away your fashion magazines and go to a Rubens exhibit or rent the Marilyn Monroe movie *Some Like It Hot* to escape the prison of petite.
- ⟲ **Skip** the super-size portion at the restaurant or take-out counter; serve your meals on smaller plates at home.
- ⟲ **Sip** on water all day long, up until an hour or two before bed.
- ⟲ **Snack** on vegetables and fruits for a great nutrition boost and natural feeling of fullness.
- ⟲ **Say no** to negative self-talk about body image and weight.
- ⟲ **Love life** in the middle of the J curve!

You can also increase your chance of weight-loss success with a self-monitoring system. Closely tracking your weight and food intake enables you to nip any gains or bad habits in the bud. You might have heard the final piece of lasting weight-loss advice from your mother: Eat breakfast. A morning meal makes the day brighter and tends to lighten up the content of the meals that follow.

Maintaining a healthy weight is a step towards a long, vibrant healthspan. The healthiest weight for you, however, probably doesn't correlate with the images that society presses upon us, and "maintaining" is a key word in the equation.

If your BMI is 27 to 29.9 with risk factors or 30 or above, ask yourself what a longer, healthier life is worth to you. Choose an evidenced-based diet that controls calories, emphasizes longevity-boosting foods, and doesn't overly restrict or promote any food or food group. Be sure of your commitment and diet sensibility. Set a reasonable weight-loss goal and take your time. If you follow the nutrition guidelines I've described in chapter 2, choosing lots of fruits and vegetables, whole grains, fish, poultry, low-fat dairy products, and moderate amounts of the good fats, you'll be surprised at how many great-tasting foods are available to you. Stick to it and you'll be establishing AgeLess habits that can last a lifetime.

If your BMI is under 27, your waistline falls into the fit zone, and you don't have medical problems that can be exacerbated by extra pounds, I urge you to put your preoccupations with weight in the past and start enjoying a guilt-free present. Stay active and watch your waistline. Meanwhile, if a partner, friend, or inner voice suggests that you aim for the figure of a fashion model, rent a Marilyn Monroe movie or take a trip to the art museum to revel in the glory of the full-figured human body.

When weighing your longevity, keep the facts in hand and don't let the notion that "thin is in" cloud your view. No matter where you currently stand on the scale, making peace with yourself is the first step to an enlightened long life.

YOUR AGELESS AGENDA
Weight

Check off each item as you achieve it:

- ☐ Body mass index (BMI) of less than 27, or less than 25 if you have two or more weight-related risk factors
- ☐ Waistline measuring less than 40 inches for men, 35 inches for women
- ☐ Regular exercise
- ☐ Freedom from fad diets
- ☐ Freedom from diet drugs (unless your BMI is 30 or above and you're taking a single prescription medication under a doctor's close supervision)
- ☐ If you're age 55 or over, minimum BMI of 20

CHAPTER 5

SLEEP

OLD SLEEP RULE	NEW SLEEP RULE
Fill your schedule and make up for lost sleep on weekends.	**#1.** Put a good night's sleep on your daily calendar.
You need less sleep as you get older.	**#2.** Make adjustments to get enough sleep throughout your life.
Insomnia and sleep problems are an inevitable part of life.	**#3.** Sleep problems can and should be treated.
A midday nap is a good rejuvenator.	**#4.** Say "no" to naps.

I BECAME A FATHER for the first time at age 49 and was 55 by the time our daughter Clare was born—so after years of good, consistent sleep that kept me at my peak, I suddenly experienced sleep deprivation. Parenthood is a tough transition anytime, but try it when you've already lived for half a century! Even now, at age 8, Clare will call for Daddy after a nightmare, so I've come up with a strategy to make sure I get the sleep I need every night. I turn in just after a last snuggle with my children and wake up before them. I make up for nighttime interruptions by sleeping a little longer in the morning to get the 8 hours I need for peak performance during the day.

Why such careful attention to my nightly z's when there's so much to be done at work and at home? Because sleep is such an important key to health and longevity. I want to do everything I can to be around for all my children's graduations and my grandkids without missing a minute of fun along the way. Spending 8 hours a night in dreamland is an investment I make in my future with my family.

WHAT'S YOUR LONGEVITY QUOTIENT?

Sleep

Take the following quiz to delve deeper into the details of your sleep LQ. Choose the one item from each checklist that describes you best and enter the points in the "Your LQ Points" column.

	Your LQ Points	Max LQ Points

Priority of Sleep

10 points: You always make time for a good night's sleep

8 points: You try to make time for a good night's sleep

6 points: You sometimes make time for a good night's sleep

4 points: You occasionally make time for a good night's sleep

0 points: You get a good night's sleep when you can fit it into your schedule   ___   **10**

Quality of Sleep

10 points: You usually get a good night's sleep and wake up refreshed

8 points: You have occasional difficulty falling or staying asleep

6 points: You have frequent difficulty falling or staying asleep

4 points: You have real trouble falling or staying asleep and occasionally need or wish for over-the-counter medications (Tylenol PM, Sominex, etc.)

2 points: You have insomnia and need prescription medications to get some sleep

0 points: You cannot sleep without prescription medications   ___   **10**

Quantity of Sleep

10 points: You usually sleep 7 or more hours a night and wake up refreshed

8 points: You usually sleep 7 or more hours a night and often wake up tired

9 points: You usually sleep 6 to 6.9 hours a night and wake up refreshed

	Your LQ Points	Max LQ Points

5 points: You usually sleep 6 to 6.9 hours a night and
often wake up tired

8 points: You usually sleep 5 to 5.9 hours a night and
wake up refreshed (really?)

2 points: You usually sleep 5 to 5.9 hours a night and
often wake up tired

0 points: You usually sleep less than 5 hours a night ___ **10**

Daytime Alertness and Naps

10 points: You usually feel refreshed and alert throughout the day

8 points: You often feel refreshed and alert but rarely all day
long, and may take or wish for a nap

5 points: You often feel somewhat sleepy and tired and take
or wish for naps

3 points: You often feel sleepy and tired and take naps as a
result

0 points: You rarely feel truly awake ___ **10**

Relaxation before Bedtime

10 points: You always relax for sleep and leave your worries
and to-do lists outside the bedroom

8 points: You usually relax for sleep and leave your worries
and to-do lists outside the bedroom

5 points: You frequently relax for sleep and leave your worries
and to-do lists outside the bedroom

3 points: You usually take your worries and to-do lists with you
into the bedroom

0 points: You always take your worries and to-do lists with you ___ **10**
into the bedroom

Bedroom As a Haven for Sleep

10 points: Your bedroom is a sleep sanctuary

8 points: You sometimes do other things in your bedroom
besides sleep (and sex)

6 points: You often do other things in your bedroom besides
sleep (and sex)

	Your LQ Points	Max LQ Points

4 points: You usually do other things in your bedroom besides sleep (and sex)

0 points: You always do other things in your bedroom besides sleep (and sex) ____ **10**

Sleep Environment

10 points: Your sleeping area is designed to minimize light and sound

8 points: You've done the best you can, but your sleeping area still admits some light and/or sound that disturbs your sleep

5 points: Your sleeping area admits some light and/or sound that disturbs your sleep and you haven't tried to fix it

3 points: You've done the best you can, but your sleeping area is still loud and/or bright and this disturbs your sleep

10 points: You don't care about light and sound in your sleeping area, but you get great sleep anyway (Are you sure you aren't fooling yourself?)

0 points: You've done nothing about light and sound in your sleeping area, and you have a hard time sleeping ____ **10**

Light Exposure

10 points: You get out into the daylight or into rooms with bright lights every day for 30 minutes or more

8 points: You get out into the daylight or into rooms with bright lights most days for 30 minutes or more

5 points: You get out into the daylight or into rooms with bright lights about every other day for 30 minutes or more

3 points: You get out into the daylight or into rooms with bright lights from time to time

0 points: You rarely or never get out into the daylight or into rooms with bright lights ____ **10**

Exercise

10 points: You engage in 30 minutes of exercise (walking, aerobics, weight training, etc.) every day

8 points: You engage in 30 minutes of exercise most days

	Your LQ Points	Max LQ Points

5 points: You engage in 30 minutes of exercise about every other day

3 points: You engage in some exercise from time to time

0 points: You rarely or never engage in exercise — **10**

Stimulants

10 points: Caffeine never keeps you awake

10 points: Caffeine keeps you awake, and you strictly avoid foods and beverages that contain it long enough before sleep to prevent this

8 points: Caffeine keeps you awake, and most of the time you avoid foods and beverages that contain it long enough before sleep

5 points: Caffeine keeps you awake, and you frequently fail to avoid foods and beverages that contain it long enough before sleep

0 points: Caffeine keeps you awake, and you fail to avoid — **10** foods and beverages that contain it long enough before sleep all or most of the time

Total — **100**

What are your sleep habits doing for your LQ? Check my diagnosis for your score below:

Total LQ Score	The Dean's Diagnosis
91–100	Rest easy; you're a super sleeper! Keep it up and consult the strategies in this chapter if sleep problems arise in the future.
81–90	You're getting adequate sleep. Sleep is on your side, but you need to move it up the priority scale to optimize your LQ.
71–80	Too tired to follow the New Rules? You need to shift priorities. Schedule more time for sleep.
61–70	Sleep deprivation danger: You may be seriously deficient in nature's original revitalizer. You can't go on this way without detriment to your longevity and health.
60 and below	Red alert! You are sleep deprived and are probably suffering the consequences and risks. Read this chapter and start following the New Rules for sleep tonight.

You've Got (Circadian) Rhythm: The Natural Cycles of Sleep

Our 24-hour sleep-wake cycle is governed by a complex sequence of hormone secretions that influence our energy level, alertness, and body temperature. These daily fluctuations are known as *circadian rhythms,* and they naturally impel us to wake with the dawn and sleep with the dusk.

The shining star in controlling your circadian rhythms is none other than the sun. When light rays hit the eye, they trigger nerve responses that send synchronizing signals to the brain. Daytime exposure to light stimulates the release of melatonin, a hormone secreted by the pineal gland, which slows you down to a state of drowsiness as night falls. This sunlight-hormone connection helps you sleep and wake in a regular daily rhythm. Night shift workers, over time, develop their own cycles in which they release melatonin in the morning so they can sleep during the day.

The Ideal Night's Sleep

What does a good night's sleep look like? In sleep labs across the country, researchers have wired subjects with electrodes to form a picture of what's called the *sleep architecture* of a healthy night of slumber. We know that only a quarter of a night's sleep is filled with dreams; the rest is divided into four stages of incrementally deeper sleep characterized by increasingly slower brain waves.

The reason researchers describe our nightly experience as sleep architecture is that it's a complex process, involving much more than closing your eyes at one end and opening them at the other. During the night, you cycle through four different sleep states. Stage one is a light doze, a dreamless state marked by theta and alpha brain waves. During stage two, or midlevel sleep, brain wave activity becomes unsettled, with irregular patterns and spikes. These irregularities smooth out as we enter stage three, a state of deep sleep, marked by long, slow delta waves. Delta wave activity increases during deepest sleep, the fourth stage of dreamless sleep that appears to be quite important to health.

After you cycle once through these four stages, you return to stage two (midlevel sleep) and then proceed to REM, the rapid eye movement stage where dreaming takes place. Brain wave activity during REM is in the beta range, a state of full alertness when you're awake,

The Sleep Cycle

Here's what a good night's sleep looks like for most adults. You can see at a glance how important the first part of the night is to deep sleep and the last to REM dream stages. Not all hours of sleep are alike, and you *do* need them all.

Stage	Type	Brain Waves	Percent of Total Sleep (hours based on an 8-hour night)
Nondreaming—75% of Total Sleep			
1	Light doze	Theta and some alpha (meditative) brain waves	5% (½ hour)
2	Midlevel sleep	Irregular, rapid activity with spikes	45% (3½ hours)
3	Deep sleep	20–50% delta waves (slow, large, regular)	12% (1 hour)
4	Deepest sleep	More than 50% delta waves	13% (1 hour)
Dreaming—25% of Total Sleep			
Rapid eye movement (REM)	Dreaming	Beta waves (similar to being awake)	25% (2 hours)

which might help explain why dreams can seem so true to life and vivid. Deep sleep (stages three and four) mostly takes place in the first third of the night and most REM time in the last third. Arise before you've put in a little over 7 hours and you may deprive yourself of your sweetest dreams!

Sleep More, Age Less

Many studies have looked at the relationship between sleep and aging, and they find that individuals who sleep an average of 7 to 9 hours a night have the longest life expectancy. This connection between lifetime and bedtime boils down to a simple ratio: Basically, we're designed to spend a third of our lives sound asleep.

Sadly—and alarmingly—getting enough sleep is a lost art. Many people consider sleep a nuisance, a brake on life in the fast lane. The National Sleep Foundation reports that the majority of Americans get less than the AgeLess recommendation of 7 to 9 hours a night. The national average clocks in at 6 hours and 54 minutes, dipping even lower during the work week. This means that nearly half of us are not getting enough sleep. The reason that most of us don't get our nightly z's is that we scacrifice them to work more, and one person in ten admitted that sleep is the first thing to go when time is tight.

Sleep is not an optional activity: It's as essential to life as water and food, a basic health requirement. So why aren't we more sleep-savvy? Probably because sleep research doesn't garner the news headlines that cancer, heart disease, and other high-profile discoveries receive. Still, sleep researchers have been quietly learning how sleep works and the wonderful benefits it offers to the body and brain.

Alert Immune Cells

In his book *The Promise of Sleep,* Dr. William Dement, founder of Stanford University's sleep disorder center, described a study showing the importance of sleep to maintaining a healthy immune system. In this British trial, researchers sent participants for a week's R&R in the English countryside, then gave them a noseful of cold virus germs and watched them for another week. Less than one in ten of the well-rested vacationers got sick, and those who did fared pretty well. The researchers determined that sleep was a key factor in fighting the cold germs, a conclusion you may have reached yourself during restful vacations and one that other studies affirm.

Conversely, a lack of sleep can unleash a hormonal assault that weakens your immune system. Your body translates sleep deprivation as stress and responds by spewing out stress hormones that can weaken immune responses, leaving you vulnerable to invading germs and antigens. If you've ever caught a cold while burning the candle at both ends, you've experienced this firsthand. The result of prolonged exposure to stress hormones is increased risk for everything from flu to heart disease, cancer, and depression. See chapter 6 for more on stress.

There's another hormonal connection between sleep and aging. During deep, delta wave sleep, adults secrete the majority of their human growth hormone (HGH). HGH is important for building bone and muscle mass and discouraging the storage of fat. HGH levels peak during adolescent years. From early adulthood and through middle age, both the amount of time spent in slow delta wave sleep and HGH levels in the bloodstream decline in tandem, suggesting a link between depth of sleep and blood levels of this youth-giving hormone. (See chapter 7 for more about HGH and the aging process and why you shouldn't take it in supplemental form.)

A study conducted in fourteen sleep labs across the country indicated that the connection between sleep and HGH secretion is strongest in men, who by age 50 are often critically short on deep sleep and as a result may lose muscle mass and gain fat. It's not yet clear how specific sleep interventions might offset age-related decline in HGH. What is clear is that HGH shots are not the solution. The apparent link between human growth hormone and slower aging has led some "antiaging" doctors to pitch growth hormone shots to their patients. I do not recommend this expensive and potentially dangerous treatment! HGH injections can have serious side effects including diabetes and carpal tunnel syndrome (a painful condition involving the swelling of tendons in your wrist). Deep sleep, however, may naturally stimulate your own HGH so that you can enjoy its youth-preserving powers without the risks and costs of supplements.

Thanks for the Memories

If you're always having trouble finding the car keys or remembering names, sleep can help you out here, too. Though scientists don't yet understand exactly how, sleep seems to help the brain consolidate and organize memory. A sleep shortage, as most of us know from experience, can significantly impair memory, and the longer you run a sleep debt, the more frequent and pervasive forgetfulness can be. Many older people mistakenly think that their memory slips stem from inevitable "aging" of our brains or even early Alzheimer's disease, when lack of sleep is actually the true culprit. Get your shut-eye, and you can thank sleep for your good memory at any age.

Good Sleep Begets Good Moods

You've probably noticed that you feel happier and more even-tempered when you're not dragging around with your eyes at half-mast. This isn't too surprising since sleep is regulated in the same brain area that controls mood, along with body temperature and hormones. This spot—the hypothalamus, located on the upper part of the brain stem—is your emotional center, and it's happiest when you've had plenty of sleep.

Mood is even more dramatically impaired by sleep deprivation than is physical performance or mental function. With six to eight percent of

the population suffering from depression and even more from dysphoria (bad moods that reduce your quality of life but don't meet clinical criteria for depression) and a majority of Americans admitting that
they don't get enough sleep, it's likely that better sleep habits could improve outlook and emotional health for many individuals. The sleep-
mood connection also seems to work the other way around. People who
feel good emotionally generally sleep better, while depression is one of
the biggest risk factors for insomnia. This apparent Catch-22 can be re-
solved by treating the sleep problem, the depression, or ideally, both.

Accident Prevention and Peak Performance

Drunk on the job? You probably wouldn't consider going to work in-
toxicated by alcohol, but showing up sleepy could impair your performance just as much. How about driving drunk? I hope you just say no
to that irresponsible act, but please also give your car keys to someone
else when you're sleep deprived. Annually, about 50,000 American auto
accidents are attributed to driving while sleepy, and more than half of
us admit to drowsy driving within the past year.

Quality sleep is critical to your life expectancy every time you drive
a car or engage in other activities with reflex-related risks. A single night
of inadequate sleep can lower your reflex time; a few in a row can make
you a serious menace to yourself and society. The media was quick to
blame the *Exxon Valdez* crash on the captain who was accused—then ac-
quited—of being drunk: In fact it was the third mate, who had slept only
six hours in the previous forty-eight, who steered the ship onto the reef.

AGELESS REWARDS
Sleep

Following the New Sleep Rules can boost your healthspan in the following ways:

- Raising human growth hormone levels
- Enhancing immunity
- Sharpening memory and mental function
- Boosting mood and easing depression
- Preventing accidents
- Improving job performance

And other major accidents from Chernobyl and Three Mile Island to the Bhopal chemical plant have been linked by investigators to sleep deprivation.

I know that for many of us getting 7 to 9 hours of sleep a night may seem like an impossible dream. There's just too much to do! Rest assured that AgeLess sleep habits will send you off to that 9:00 A.M. meeting or soccer match with bright eyes and energy to burn. Though getting enough sleep may leave you a little less time to get everything done tomorrow, you'll probably do what you have to do more efficiently. Make getting enough sleep a priority.

NEW SLEEP RULE #1:
PUT A GOOD NIGHT'S SLEEP
ON YOUR DAILY CALENDAR

It sounds obvious, but it's advice many of us need: You need to set aside the time to sleep. Just as you make time for work, family, play, exercise, community, spirituality, and friends, you need to write sleep into your

AgeLess Sleep Journal

Night	Bedtime (under the covers)	Time to Fall Asleep*	Estimated Asleep Time	Estimated Time Awake during Night
Example	10:30 P.M.	Medium	10:45 P.M.	30 min
Sunday				
Monday				
Tuesday				
Wednesday				
Thursday				
Friday				
Saturday				

Note any sleep-related factors, such as naps, caffeine or other stimulants, illness or injury, pain, allergies, hot flashes, medications, or changes in schedule or routines.

schedule. A study in Sweden found that of the people who suffered from sleep deprivation, only half had actual difficulty sleeping. The other half simply didn't allow themselves a full night's sleep.

Sleep researchers use the term *sleep debt* for the amount of sleep you "owe" in order to return to baseline health and performance. The short-term debt you run after a late night followed by an early morning can make the next day much less productive and pleasant. It's how much debt you accumulate over time that matters most to your healthspan. There's a mechanism in your brain that compares the sleep you get to the sleep you need. You can build up a huge sleep debt slowly and imperceptibly over weeks and months. The resulting stress to the body and brain may contribute to the development of depression and the condition called chronic fatigue syndrome, to name just two of many possible health consequences.

Assess Yourself: Your AgeLess Sleep Journal

You probably know what your bank balance is—but when was the last time you checked on your sleep deficit? My students are often sur-

Week of _____

Time Arose from Bed	Total Hours Asleep**	Wanted more?	Quality of Sleep***
6:30 A.M.	7:15 hr	Yes, a little	Good

*Fast: a few minutes; Medium: up to 15 minutes; Slow: more than 15 minutes
**Total hours asleep = Estimated asleep time to time arose from bed minus estimated time awake during night
***Excellent, Good, Fair, or Poor

Shift Workers Need Sleep, Too!

Getting enough sleep is even harder for people who work at night, especially if they have frequent shift changes. This doesn't mean shift workers should settle for less sleep. Use the sleep journal and information in this chapter to figure out how much sleep you need, and make sure you get it. Try blackout drapes to create nighttime sleeping conditions during daylight hours.

prised when they compare their perceptions of their sleep habits to hard reality.

To assess your current sleep adequacy, use the AgeLess Sleep Journal on pages 150 and 151 to track your actual sleeping patterns for a week. Continue keeping your sleep journal until you meet your personal requirements with the help of the strategies in this chapter. You can photocopy this form or keep your own log in a notebook.

Larks and Owls

As with so many things, no two people are identical when it comes to their sleep patterns and needs. First, there's the question of night owls versus morning larks. Some people are ready to turn in long before Letterman and happily bound out of bed at first light, while others experience a surge of late-night energy and would rather stay up late and sleep in. How much of this is habit or due to genetic differences in circadian rhythms we don't know, but needless to say, larks don't do well on the night shift, or vice versa.

If you have trouble staying up late or feel cranky or tired during the day, deep down inside you may be a lark! For millennia, people rose and retired with the sun; a few members of the privileged class could burn expensive midnight lamp oil. Only in the past century has the invention of electric light made staying up late an easy option. Owls take note that evidence shows exposure to bright daylight improves sleep and mood. Sleeping away daylight hours may not be the best way to ensure your health and well-being.

If you're hooked on the *Tonight* show, *Monday Night Football*, the movie of the week, or any other television program that keeps you up past your bedtime, I recommend that you use a VCR, Replay-TV, or TiVo to record your favorite show and play it back the next day at 7 instead of 11. You'll be able to fast-forward through the commercials!

The AgeLess Sleep Calculator

For reasons we haven't completely unraveled, individual sleeps needs are different within the seven to nine hour range. Resist the temptation to make do with seven hours simply because it suits your busy schedule.

Here's how to determine your personal nightly sleep requirement. Take a week to experiment. Assess how you feel each morning when you get up. Do you keep pounding your clock radio's snooze button, or do you have that refreshed "all's well with the world" feeling? Follow the instructions below and record your results in your sleep journal.

Need More Sleep?

If after a normal night's sleep you still want more or you feel sleepy during the day:

1. Go to bed 15 minutes earlier tonight or get up 15 minutes later tomorrow.

2. Continue to add a 15-minute block of sleep time for each of the following nights until you wake up refreshed and satisfied. That's your optimal sleep allowance.

Need Less Sleep?

If you seem to be getting plenty of sleep or are waking up before your alarm:

1. Go to bed 15 minutes later tonight or set your alarm for 15 minutes earlier tomorrow.

2. Continue to subtract a 15-minute block of sleep time for each of the following nights until you wake up tired or get sleepy during the day.

3. Add back 15 minutes. That's your optimal sleep allowance.

MAKE ADJUSTMENTS TO GET ENOUGH SLEEP THROUGHOUT YOUR LIFE

When I was a medical intern in my mid-twenties, I could fall asleep anytime, anywhere. Once on daily rounds, during a discussion of one of my patients, two of my professors lapsed into a long debate over a particular aspect of the case. I was dead tired, but it wasn't considered proper for the interns to sit down, so I propped myself up against a podium and tried to follow the scholarly discourse with close attention and proper respect. When it was over, my professors found me fast asleep, head resting on the podium, chin gently cupped in my hand.

Med school was like that, and still is, showing that even the most health-conscious among us don't give sleep it's due as a component of health. Many of us started burning the midnight oil in college, studying for that final or finishing up that paper, figuring we'd make up for it the next day. We got away with it, then, didn't we? Well, folks, if you're over 30, those days are gone. Though you need as much sleep as ever, your ability to get it diminishes as nature begins to take back the gift of sleep she bequeathed in youth. Natural changes in brain wave activity begin to alter the shape of the sleep architecture. You spend less time in restorative deep sleep (stages three and four) and your first round of REM dreamtime shortens. It takes longer to fall asleep and stress, the sound of traffic noise, or even the glow of your clock's digital display may be enough to wake you. Your circadian rhythms can also change, waking you up earlier and making it hard to get back to sleep. If you're like most people, you ignore these developments, suffering through sleepy days for so long that you forget what full alertness feels like.

Insomnia also is a very common complaint during menopause. Among the culprits that interfere with sleep are night sweats, which are caused by a malfunction in the body's thermostat. These bouts of excessive sweating are accompanied by elevated heart rate and can awaken some women many times a night. (See chapter 7 for more about menopause.)

The first step in responding to these changes is to understand that even though sleep does slip away with age, there are things you can do to get it back.

NEW SLEEP RULE #3:
SLEEP PROBLEMS CAN AND SHOULD BE TREATED

Forty million Americans have some trouble sleeping, so if you're one of them, you're hardly alone. In fact, sleep is so crucial to health and elusive to so many people that there's a whole new medical specialty known as sleep medicine. Organizations such as the American Academy of Sleep Medicine, the National Sleep Foundation, and the National Center on Sleep Disorders Research are dedicated to the research and treatment of sleep disorders.

What to Expect When . . .

Sleeping patterns change throughout your life, often making sleep harder to get—but still necessary.

- ⑥ **Childhood:** Deep sleep time! Most of the night is spent sound asleep (stages three and four), and you get plenty of vivid REM dreams, making sleep as refreshing as it is necessary to rapid development and growth.
- ⑥ **Teens:** A precipitous drop in deep sleep corresponds with the maturing of the body and brain.
- ⑥ **Twenties:** Deep stage three and four sleep begins a long, slow decline that lasts through middle age. You're probably too excited about being twentysomething to notice.
- ⑥ **Thirties:** Start counting sheep. Shifts in brain waves, busy schedules, and lack of exercise can affect quantity and quality of sleep just when its rejuvenating powers are most welcome.
- ⑥ **Forties and fifties:** For women, menopause brings hot flashes, soaked sheets, and frequent awakenings at night. Some people start to develop conditions that can disturb sleep such as cardiovascular and lung disease, arthritis, and enlarged prostate. As deep sleep time continues to diminish, making an effort to get enough sleep becomes critical.
- ⑥ **Sixties and seventies:** Health conditions, medications, lack of bright light exposure, and weakening of the circadian rhythms are primary culprits in nixing a good night's sleep, often leading to a negative (but preventable!) cycle of daytime napping and nighttime sleeplessness.
- ⑥ **Eighties:** Less mobility and activity can lead to further daylight deprivation, causing the circadian rhythms of many confined seniors to go so far out of cycle that they sleep during the day and stay awake all night.

Finding it hard to wake up in the morning and daytime sleepiness are the most obvious signs of a sleep shortage. Dropping off in front of the TV, drowsiness during long meetings, needing lots of coffee to stay awake, and droopy eyes while driving are other telling signs. Sleeping in on weekends may seem like a luxury, but it should serve as a wake-up call: You're not getting enough sleep during the week! Do you nap during the day or wish you could? Consider this a reminder that you were sleep deprived last night and possibly nights before. Do you have bad moods, trouble concentrating, memory slips? These are potential clues pointing to low sleep levels.

Insomnia

Insomnia is defined as difficulty falling asleep or staying asleep that results in tiredness the next day—but insomnia is not a disease that causes sleeplessness. It's a symptom of physical, psychological, or environmental factors that are keeping you awake. If you've despaired that you "have" insomnia, it may be reassuring to learn that many of its causes can be addressed with simple behavioral and environmental measures.

Although there is a continuum of sleep problems, some sleep experts divide insomnia into two main categories, transient and chronic. Transient insomnia is a period of troubled sleeping that lasts up to fourteen nights, while chronic insomnia is sleeplessness that extends for more than two weeks. Anyone can have transient insomnia triggered by a stressful event; for instance, the national incidence of sleep problems shot up after the terrorist attacks of September 11, 2001. Good sleepers generally return to normal when their stress subsides, but the estimated five to ten million Americans with persistent difficulty sleeping may not. Transient and chronic insomnia can combine as a syndrome of intermittent periods of sleeplessness over time, and this may actually be the most common type of sleep trouble.

The main causes of insomnia are emotions—stress, worry, or excitement—schedule or time zone changes, and a poor sleeping environment. Some highly alert people are more sensitive to these variables than others, and we all experience different degrees of such disruptions at different times of life.

I had never had much trouble sleeping until my children were born. Not only do I have a sleep-friendly constitution, but I've long known how sleep patterns change with age and have always taken measures to make sure that I got enough. Now, I've simply added new tactics to counter the pressures of parenthood. My coauthor, Elizabeth, on the other hand, has had a hard time getting sleep since she was a child. Though she's more than twenty years younger than I am, she has to pay much more attention to her good sleep habits than I do. Fortunately, she reports better sleep than ever since working on this chapter!

Other Sleep Problems

In addition to age-related sleep changes are actual sleep disorders—physiological sleep disruptions that aren't considered normal. The two conditions of greatest concern to doctors and sleepers are sleep-disordered breathing and restless legs syndrome. Diseases such as arthritis, fibromyalgia, chronic pain, asthma or other pulmonary disease, esophageal reflux, irritable bowel syndrome, thyroid conditions, peptic ulcer disease, dementia, prostate enlargement, and urinary incontinence can also disrupt your sleep cycle.

Sleep-disordered breathing. Also known as sleep apnea, this condition occurs when your body briefly forgets to or can't breathe while you sleep, causing you to wake up perhaps countless times a night. The most common type of sleep apnea occurs when the muscles of the airway get so relaxed that they partly or completely collapse, obstructing the passage of air to your lungs. Obesity is the primary risk factor for this type of sleep apnea, and the symptoms can be as obvious as loud snoring or as subtle as daytime sleepiness. Few people know that they're waking up gasping for air many times a night, but the stress on your body and distress to the person sleeping next to you can be severe. The risks of sleep apnea run from sleep deprivation to sudden death—so if you or your partner suspects you might have this condition, see your doctor. It can be successfully treated by devices that keep the air flowing to your lungs with positive airway pressure or relieved by surgery that widens the airway passage.

Restless legs syndrome. Restless legs syndrome is characterized by periodic leg movements, which can be as often as every 20 to 40 seconds. Like sleep apnea, these movements can wake you up again and again, and you are often the last to know. Your partner is probably all too aware, though! As many as 35 percent of people 65 and older may suffer from periodic limb movements.

If you think you might have either of these disorders or suffer from one of the diseases I mentioned above, talk to your doctor about how your condition is affecting your sleep. Some simple measures such as those described below can help counter the sleep disturbances posed by medical conditions.

   ⑥ **Arthritis:** Take your pain medication at bedtime. Use extra pillows to cushion painful joints (knees, hips, shoulders).

- ⊚ **Esophageal reflux:** Take antacid medication at bedtime. Raise the head of your bed or use several pillows to elevate your head and neck, reducing reflux pressure up the esophagus.
- ⊚ **Heart and lung diseases:** Raise the head of your bed or use several pillows to elevate your head and neck, enabling better circulation and breathing.
- ⊚ **Prostate enlargement:** Avoid drinking liquids for 2 hours prior to bedtime. Empty your bladder right before going to bed.
- ⊚ **Urinary incontinence:** Avoid drinking liquids for 2 hours prior to bedtime. Empty your bladder right before going to bed. Use absorbent pads or garments for added security and peace of mind.

DR. WILLIAM DEMENT'S

Top 10 Tips to Beat Sleep Debt

William Dement, M.D., Ph.D., is founder of the world's first sleep disorders center at Stanford University, a Stanford professor, founder of the American Sleep Disorders Association, and a best-selling author. Dr. Dement explains that we now know that lost sleep accumulates as a debt—and you're borrowing against your performance and health. The two main causes of sleep debt accumulation are inadequate amounts of sleep and undiagnosed or untreated sleep disorders. Use Dr. Dement's top 10 tips to stay debt-free.

1. **Track how you feel all day.** The best way to evaluate the health and quality of your sleep for yourself is to pay close attention to the way you feel throughout the entire day. Any drowsiness in the daytime means you have a fairly large or very large sleep debt. On the other hand, if you're wide awake, clearheaded, cheerful, and full of energy all day long, you don't have a sleep problem no matter what you think.
2. **Identify any specific sleep disorder you might have.** Sleep disorders account for a full 90 percent of all insomnia and/or daytime fatigue problems.
3. **Define the problem by pinpointing the nature of your insomnia.** Do you experience trouble falling asleep or staying asleep? Are you waking up too often, too early, or a combination? How often do you have trouble sleeping? How severe is it on a typical night? Understanding the problem can help you devise a strategy for solving it. (Use the sleep journal in this chapter to implement this tip.)
4. **Practice good sleep hygiene.** Small changes in your sleep habits can make a big difference.

AgeLess Tactics for a Good Night's Sleep

Whether you face age-related sleep challenges, occasional or frequent insomnia, a high-stress schedule, or a medical condition that keeps you awake, there are many things you can do to get better sleep. You may think you've heard all the advice on sound sleep before—don't read in bed, cut the caffeine, and so on. But have you? Few people know the facts and even fewer put them to work. If we all ran the rest of our schedules in the pell-mell way we handle our sleep needs, little would ever get done. But just as you keep a calendar and balance your checkbook, you can adopt a few simple tactics to safeguard your sleep.

Catch some rays. The biological clock in your brain that controls

---

5. **Deal with your bed partner.** Does he or she snore, kick, or engage in other disturbing behaviors? Loud snoring usually means everyone in the bedroom is losing sleep.

6. **Make sleep easy.** Though people with a huge sleep debt can sleep anytime, anywhere, if you're getting enough sleep or close to it, you'll naturally have lighter sleep and be more sensitive to discomfort, including a bad mattress.

7. **Know what time it is on your biological clock** and sleep when it works best for your own body. Many people try to live out of sync with their circadian clocks, which control alertness levels. If this alerting influence occurs earlier than you plan to arise, you'll have early morning wakeups. Late alerting can lead to sleep-onset insomnia. Adjusting your schedule to your body's clock can make sleep easier.

8. **Check your breathing.** While you sleep, your breathing should be quiet and effortless, or as quiet and effortless as possible. Labored or noisy breathing could be disturbing your sleep.

9. **Don't be afraid of prescription hypnotics.** Recently marketed sleep medications are entirely safe, very effective, have minimal side effects, and are nonaddictive. If sleeping pills are the answer to obtaining adequate restorative sleep and being wide awake and energetic all day long, there is no reason to choose to be miserable. If you need insulin, you take it. Likewise with sleep medicine.

10. **When should you or your bed partner consult a sleep specialist?** Answer: when a troublesome problem related to sleep does not respond to sleep strategies or gets worse.

Discover more about the fascinating area of sleep research and what you can do to reduce your sleep debt in Dr. Dement's book *The Promise of Sleep* (Dell).

your circadian rhythms is governed by light, making the rays of the sun the most basic and natural sleep treatment you can get. You may have noticed how a day sailing, playing golf, or skiing outdoors can brighten your mood and lead to a lovely night's sleep. This is because your eye translates light into messages to the brain that can help improve mood and set your sleep cycle. A winter day, on the other hand, in which you go to work in the dark, spend the day in dim office light, and return home after nightfall, can turn your mood gloomy and result in a restless night's sleep.

Our body's circadian rhythms start to weaken with age, requiring more light to keep them synchronized just as you're likely to get less— first because you're so busy working, later because you may not leave the house as much. The pattern of melatonin secreation changes. Instead of a spike of excretion at 10:00 P.M., the peak is dampened and spread over many hours. People in nursing homes get very little bright light, and their rhythms can become so confused that they sleep during the day and stay awake all night.

To easily improve your night's sleep, open the curtains during the day, install a bright light at work or wherever you spend the most time, and get out in natural sunlight as often as you can (with sunscreen and sunglasses on, of course). Take a walk at lunch. Position your desk near a window. Take your morning jog outdoors instead of on a treadmill inside. If it's too cold or inclement outside, choose a treadmill next to a window at the gym or do your home workout in the sunniest spot in the house. Just like your skin, your eyes can soak up the sun's rays even on cloudy days.

You can buy special high-watt lamps designed for light therapy. For some people who live in far northern regions, this is the only way to get enough light in the winter to regularize sleep and prevent seasonal affective disorder (SAD), otherwise known as the winter blues, which can come with light deprivation. Talk with your doctor before buying such a light to ensure that you use it safely and effectively.

Get hot. One of the best ways to sleep peacefully through the still of the night is to get moving during the day. Exercise, particularly movement that heats up the body enough to make you break a sweat, helps people fall asleep faster, sleep longer, and wake up less. Most importantly, exercise increases the quantity of deep, slow-wave sleep. Body temperature significantly decreases when you sleep, and this may actually trigger the onset of sleep. Experts think that in addition to releasing tension and promoting overall health, exercise may abet sleep by raising body temperature and exaggerating the subsequent drop at bedtime. The key is to exercise every day to enjoy optimal sleep every night.

Timing also counts. The earlier in the day you exercise, the greater the improvement in slow-wave sleep that night. There's another sleep-related reason to exercise early. Working out within as much as 6 hours before bedtime can stimulate your body enough to interfere with sleep. That means that the workout you get from an evening salsa session may not help your insomnia. There's one nighttime workout that might serve as just the sleep medication you need: sex. This form of exercise seems to serve as a soporific for many of us.

Another way to change body temperature to help you drop off to sleep is a hot bath, Jacuzzi, or shower right before bed. If you have dry skin, apply moisturizing lotion after your bath so itchy skin doesn't plague you in the middle of the night.

Don't forget to exercise your mind, too. Many jobs make you work up plenty of mental sweat during the day, but if you're retired or not very challenged at work, turn off the TV and read a good book, have a scintillating conversation, attend a social event, do a crossword puzzle, or play a challenging game such as bridge or chess. Make mental exercise and stimulating exchange with others a daily habit so your mind will be tired each night. As with physical exercise, be sure to allow enough time to unwind between revving up your brain and going to bed.

Make your bedroom a sleep sanctuary. Start by checking out the windows—do your curtains shut out all light? If not, go to the linen store, hold different drapes up to the light to see how much seeps through, then choose the one that blocks light best. You can even get special blackout drapes if you're very sensitive to light. Buy the best quality you can afford. This investment will pay off immediately and beats shelling out money for sleeping pills any day or night!

Next, look at all the light sources in your bedroom. The worst offender may be your alarm clock. Some LED displays emit enough light to fool you into thinking it's morning all night long. Each time you wake up to look at the clock it worries your tired mind about how late or early it is—stimulation you don't need. If you have a lighted clock, turn the display at an angle so you can still see the time but most of the light is directed away from the eyes. Try to break the habit of checking the time during the night. The alarm will alert you soon enough.

Likewise, avoid using a night-light in your bedroom or leaving a door open to a lit hallway if you can. Some people appreciate a little help navigating the path to the bathroom, especially seniors. Buy the dimmest nightlight you can find and place it as far from your bed as possible. Or get a motion-activated night-light that will go on only when you get out of bed. Better still, keep a small flashlight on your night table.

A sleeping mask is essential for night shift workers who must sleep during the day and is also helpful when your best efforts can't eliminate light from your environment. Simple and cheap, this solution will keep the light out of your eyes.

Managing noise is next. People often insist that sound doesn't bother their sleep, that they can get used to anything. Research shows otherwise. A study of people who lived near a noisy airport found that they averaged an hour less sleep each night than those living in quiet neighborhoods. If street noise is a problem in your area, look for drapes that block sound as well as light, and add carpeting and wall hangings to help absorb the sound. If your neighbor likes to blast his stereo late at night, try to negotiate a schedule that works for everyone. If you can't eliminate environmental sounds, try soft relaxing music, a fan, or a white noise machine. Look for the pure white noise machines used by medical professionals, which offer a constant sound environment, rather than the synthesized nature sound machines found in department stores. Keep a set of polyurethane or wax earplugs on your bedside table. Whether you use them when a partner snores or during the neighbor's late night parties, they're a great insurance policy at home and on the road. I always travel with earplugs as a defense against traffic noise and loud activities in adjacent hotel rooms.

If you have a TV in your bedroom, move it! Watching television in bed deconditions your mind from sleep and overstimulates the body and brain, and falling asleep with it on guarantees that you'll wake up later to turn it off.

As for that lumpy mattress and bedraggled pillow: Pamper yourself with proper bedding and see how easy sleep can be. I'm often astonished by how many supposedly poor sleepers suffer from little more than the princess and the pea syndrome. Go to a good bed store and bounce around. If money is a factor, remember that your comfort is the bottom line. The mattress salesperson will remind you that spending an extra $500 for a quality mattress that lasts 10 years comes out to a mere 14 cents a night. If you'd pay $3 for a fancy coffee to wake you up, wouldn't a few pennies spent to get a good night's sleep make sense?

Temperature is another hot topic. Many people find that they sleep better in a cool room, perhaps because a drop in body temperature serves as a trigger to sleep. A cooler room is also more comfortable during the night sweats of menopause. But feeling cold can keep you awake, so don't go overboard. Experiment with different settings on the thermostat, number and type of blankets, opening or closing windows, and using a fan (a ceiling fan is nice because it doesn't blow directly on you). If your sleeping partner has a different temperature threshold, consider an electric blanket with dual controls. Do what it takes to make your bedroom feel just right.

Finally, keep your worries out of the bedroom. You have plenty of waking hours in other rooms of the house to devote to the cares of the world. Your bedroom should be a worry-free retreat, a rejuvenating haven where you can stop doing and simply be—so clear out all the files and clutter, the piles of paper and reminders of responsibilities and pro-jects. Your only job here is to sleep and relax.

Relax already! We live in a world of stress and information overload, and unwinding after a busy day can be a big challenge. Still, you can learn to relax to a sleep-inducing state and rely on this ability for the rest of your life.

Nature gave us a highly attuned alertness system so that we could react to defend ourselves from predators. You've probably heard plenty about this stress response—a series of hormone secretions that quickens your heart rate and breathing, boosts brain wave activity, tenses muscles, and slows down immune response and digestion to free up energy for fighting or fleeing. The trouble is that these days, the stress response can be evoked by anything from a traffic snarl to a slow Internet connection, and stress hormones from daytime pressures can still be circulating in your bloodstream when it's time to go to sleep, keeping you on high alert.

Fortunately, researchers have found that relaxation techniques have quantifiable effects. They can stem the secretion of stress hormones, slow brain waves and calm mental activity, reduce heart and respiratory rate, and relax muscles. All these changes are gateways to sleep.

Relaxation is so important to round-the-clock wellness that we discuss it in more depth in chapter 6. Read the techniques described on page 182. Try them first during the day, when you don't have the pressure of trying to fall asleep, and keep practicing them until you can attain a relaxed feeling whenever you need it. Once you reach that level of comfort, use these relaxation exercises just before or after getting into bed to transition into a sleep state, as well as anytime you awaken during the night.

Practice good sleep hygiene. You might associate hygiene more with caring for your teeth than with going to sleep, but good sleep hygiene—a set of habits that promote sound sleep—is especially important for people with sleeping problems. Based on behavioral conditioning and the physiology of sleep, these techniques can help overcome insomnia and make sleep as automatic as brushing your teeth. Here are the key practices that support sweet dreams:

⊚ **Keep to a schedule.** Go to bed at the same time each night and get up at the same time each morning, including weekends. If your schedule changes, gradually adjust your routine over a number of days to give your body time to adapt.

AGELESS TIP

Leave Your Worries at the Bedroom Door

Every night when you walk through your bedroom door, take a few deep breaths, relax those taut muscles, and let your mind go clear. Schedule a "worry time" during the day, and then forbid them to reoccur at night. It might sound silly, but it works for many people.

If items for your to-do list spring from your subconscious mind all night long, keep a small pad and pen by the bed so you can jot them down and get right back to sleep. Use a small flashlight or pen with a built-in light so you don't have to turn on a lamp.

---

⑥ **Go to bed to sleep.** Don't let yourself fall asleep in front of the TV or reading in your favorite chair. Be firm with yourself. Don't lie down to watch TV if you know you'll drift off to sleep.

⑥ **Use the bed only for sleep.** That's right, no more reading in bed. Create a cozy nook in another room for reading and watching TV if you're used to doing these things in the comfort of bed. Exception: Amorous activities are allowed.

⑥ **Don't nap.** My advice is to not take naps, but there are times when a nap may be an important safety measure (if you feel drowsy and must drive, for instance). You may also be a good sleeper who welcomes a nap after being kept up at night by a sick child or car alarm. But keep it under an hour and finish by 3:00 P.M.

⑥ **Limit caffeine.** If you're sensitive to caffeine, set your personal cutoffs for quantity and time. People have different responses, so use your sleep journal to track yours. You may find that you can enjoy a few cups of coffee as long as you stop by 4:00 P.M., for instance, or that you need to stick to one cup and drink it before noon in order to get a good night's sleep.

⑥ **Avoid nicotine** close to bedtime and during the night, since it is a stimulant.

⑥ **Finish vigorous exercise** by 2 to 6 hours before bedtime; use your sleep journal to find your own window of time. Stretching or yoga is fine and may help you to relax.

⑥ **Don't eat a heavy meal** right before bed. If you're hungry, try a light snack such as a piece of toast with honey, or better still, a few slices of turkey or a glass of warm milk about an hour before bedtime. Both contain L-tryptophan, a wonderful natural sleep enhancer. Milk must be heated to make the tryptophan active.

⑥ **Stop drinking liquids** an hour or so before bed to prevent trips to the bathroom in the middle of the night.

Take a time-out. What if all your good sleep hygiene habits fail to send you off to slumberland? That's the time to take a time-out from bed.

If you don't fall asleep after 15 minutes of trying (or of waking up

Caffeine Undercover

Most of us know that tea, coffee, and Coca-Cola are packed with caffeine, but did you know that Dr Pepper and Mountain Dew are also laced with the eye-opening stimulant? A slice of chocolate cake may also keep you awake, since that ambrosial food, chocolate, is full of a caffeine-related compound. If you have trouble sleeping, watch out for all stimulants and observe your personal limits.

in the middle of the night), get out of bed and do something quiet in another room with a light on—read, listen to soft music or a book on tape, knit, or write. Return to bed only when you feel drowsy. Repeat this time-out for every 15-minute period of wakefulness. Get up at the usual time the following morning.

You may be tired on the days following time-outs, but you would be anyway—and your breaks from the bedroom yield two lasting benefits. First, you follow your circadian rhythms so that tomorrow night's weariness will promote sleep. Secondly, just saying no to lying awake in bed conditions your body and brain to sleep when you're there—a strong behavioral link that you may never have made before. Be cautious if you're driving or engaging in other activities requiring quick reflexes on the day after a wakeful night.

Research has found that this simple wakefulness break routine can help you overcome even chronic insomnia, provided there's no underlying medical disorder. It may take up to a few weeks to break your old pattern and establish a new one, but the effort and the short-term low energy days will pay off in a better sleep that can last for a (longer) lifetime.

Cigarettes and Sleep

If you smoke, you may find that sleep deprivation deepens your reliance on cigarettes, and smoking can make sleep problems worse. If you commonly reach for a cigarette to perk up, try getting enough sleep instead. Avoid smoking at bedtime, and *never* smoke in bed. Nicotine is a stimulant: It can keep you awake, and bedroom fires pose a serious threat to your longevity.

NEW SLEEP RULE #4:
SAY "NO" TO NAPS

Naps are necessary for babies and tempting to grownups after a nice big lunch. Naps are also sometimes promoted as a productivity tool, with some corporations installing special nap rooms where sleepy employees

Sleep Stoppers and Keepers

How many saboteurs threaten your good night's sleep? Fight back with these AgeLess sleep solutions.

Sleep Stoppers	Sleep Keepers
Overwork, stress	Keep your work and to-do list out of your bedroom, schedule sleep in your calendar, and use relaxation techniques at stressful times and before bed.
Young children	Match your sleep schedule as closely to theirs as you can. Resist the urge to stay up long after their bedtime to catch up on tasks; you can get a jump on those jobs tomorrow! Go to bed early so there's time to make up for lost sleep in the morning if they wake you up during the night.
Early awakening	Get out into bright light every day. Do not nap. If necessary, go to bed earlier.
Shift work	Sound- and lightproof your bedroom. Do everything you can to stick to your sleeping schedule, including on weekends and holidays.
Partner who snores or other noise	Use earplugs and/or a white noise machine. Have your partner visit a sleep clinic to try antisnoring approaches such as adhesive strips, pillows, dental appliances, and surgery if indicated and all else fails.
Caffeine overload	Avoid caffeinated coffee, tea, soft drinks, and chocolate for several hours before bedtime.
Nonrestful sleep environment	Take a weekend to make your bedroom conducive to sleep, clearing out distractions and taking measures to cut light and noise.
Hot flashes	Consider treatments (see chapter 7).
Late night television or Internet surfing	Set a cut-off time and stick to it, saving any late show you don't want to miss with a VCR, TiVo, or ReplayTV. Dim the lights and play soft music to slowly lower your stimulus level as you prepare for bed.

can drop in for a snooze. Is this new nap consciousness good news for health-enhancing sleep?

For many people the answer is no, especially if you have any sort of sleep problems. Naps can upset your body clock, keeping you awake and alert at bedtime. And the payoff isn't much. A nap is too short to cycle you through all the deep sleep and dream states you need to realize the benefits of sleep. Though you may feel temporarily refreshed afterward, a nap just slaps a Band-Aid on your sleep debt. At the end of the day, you lose.

If the threat of disturbing your natural sleep patterns isn't enough to keep you from nodding off during the day, how about the risk of sudden death? Researchers have found a correlation between afternoon naps and increased mortality in older people. Yes, the simple act of awakening may be hazardous to your health, causing an abrupt rise in blood pressure and heart rate that scientists think may trigger a heart attack or stroke. Waking up still beats the alternative, but why run this risk more than once a day?

Needing to nap is a sign that you aren't getting enough sleep at night. Fix the problem at the source, and for daytime refreshment try the meditation techniques covered in chapter 6.

I make two exceptions to the no-naps rule. First, if you feel sleepy and must engage in an activity requiring quick reflexes such as driving, a nap could be key to your life expectancy. Secondly, if you have no problem with insomnia but have lost some sleep due to an unexpected event—a child's nightmare, a house alarm going off at midnight—you can take a nap to make it up the following day. I do this myself when one of my kids is sick and has kept me up for a few hours the night before. Still, naps should always be considered only a short-term solution to an emergency sleep loss and are only suitable for people without sleeping problems.

Doc, What Can I Take?

In the quest for sleep, many people seek solutions they can swallow and many doctors are all too willing to comply. However, sleeping pills should be a measure of last resort. In this you'll see that my views are somewhat more cautious then those of my esteemed colleague William Dement (see page 158). This is because in my experience addiction to sleep medications is a common problem among the elderly. However, if used judiciously, pharmaceuticals (particularly the new generation of pills you'll find in the chart on page page 170) can offer relief for the occasional very bad night and help break patterns of sleeplessness for people with serious sleeping problems.

Over-the-Counter Options

The first formulations to try are over-the-counter sleep aids, which have far fewer side effects and risks than prescription medications do. Most of the popular ones contain the antihistamines diphenhydramine or doxylamine as their main active ingredient and should not be taken by individuals with enlarged prostates, glaucoma, or respiratory problems. The table below provides an overview of some of these products and their active ingredients.

Prescription Sleeping Pills

If over-the-counter sleep aids fail, you might want to talk with your doctor about prescription drugs. No prescription sleep medication comes without side effects and tradeoffs. The long-lasting pills (10 hours or more) can leave you with a hangover, drowsiness, and fatigue on the following day, while short-acting drugs can cause rebound insomnia after you stop taking them. Given a choice, I recommend the short-acting medications (2 to 5 hours) zaleplon (Sonata) and

Over-the-Counter Sleep Aids

Though they go by many names, most over-the-counter sleep aids are similar in effectiveness and ingredients.

Product	Active Ingredients
Excedrin PM	Diphenhydramine and acetaminophen
Tylenol PM	Diphenhydramine and acetaminophen
Benadryl	Diphenhydramine
Compoz	Diphenhydramine
Nytol	Diphenhydramine
Sominex	Diphenhydramine
Unisom	Doxylamine

Prescription Sleep Medications

Here are some of the popular prescription sleeping pills along with their speed of onset, how long they last, possible problems in taking them, and their prices. The two current bestsellers are zolpidem (Ambien) and zaleplon (Sonata), which are relatively short acting and effective.

Trade Name	Generic Name	Puts You to Sleep	Lasts	Contraindications	Price*
Sonata	Zaleplon	Fast	Short time	Liver problems	$56
Prosom	Estazolam	Fast	Long time	Being treated for AIDS	$24
Dalmane	Flurazepam	Fast	Very long time	Being treated for AIDS Should not be taken by seniors	$11
Doral	Quazepam	Fast	Very long time	Additional monitoring may be required if you're taking clozapine, disulfiram, rifampin, nefazodone, or seizure medications. Should not be taken by seniors	$83
Halcion	Triazolam	Intermediate	Short time	Drinking grapefruit juice	$16
Ambien	Zolpidem	Intermediate	Short time	Taking ritonavir (Kaletra and Norvir)	$57
Restoril	Temazepam	Slow	Long time	Additional monitoring may be required if you're taking clozapine, disulfiram, or seizure medications. Seniors should take this drug cautiously.	$118

* Approximate November 2002 prices for 30 pills of smallest dose available (generic if available)

zolpidem (Ambien), which have less hangover effect. Cost also varies widely among sleeping pills, as you can see in the table below. Your physician can advise you on medications to address your personal sleep needs.

The single most important thing to remember about sleeping pills is that you should never take them for more than a few days at a time. Dependence can soon lead to addiction, and this is a sleep problem you definitely don't want to have.

Natural Remedies

The best natural sleep remedies are the ones described in this chapter. The two most popular entries in this category are melatonin and valerian root.

Since melatonin is the main hormone involved in sending us to sleep, it seems to follow that it would be an effective soporific—but research hasn't been able to support this claim. From tests on space shuttle astronauts to lab experiments monitoring slow wave sleep and unwanted wake-ups, we can't seem to find any significant sleep benefits from melatonin. Furthermore, there are no long-term studies on the safety of supplemental melatonin, and hormones are powerful substances. There may also be risks in taking melatonin over an extended period of time.

Valerian root is an herb sold as a sleep aid. Though some people report easier sleep after taking valerian, objective measures of patients' brain waves, which quantify actual sleep time and stages, have failed to find that valerian assists in falling asleep faster, waking up less, or returning to sleep sooner after nighttime awakenings. The professional consensus is that valerian's primary effect may be on your perception of how fast you fall asleep, and though perception can be a powerful force, it doesn't deliver the benefits of sleep itself. New Rules recommendation: Leave valerian in the vial unless we learn something vital and new.

L-tryptophan, a compound that influences neurotransmitter activity in the brain, was widely used in supplement form as a natural sleep remedy until a number of people died after taking contaminated supplements. Since the risk of contamination is inherent to the manufac-

The Pill for Weekend Partiers (and Weary Travelers)

One thing melatonin does seem to do is help reset a sleep schedule disrupted by jet lag, shift work, or staying up late on the weekend. A study at the Sleep Disorders Center in New York City has shown that popping a melatonin pill late Sunday afternoon after a weekend of burning midnight oil can help you slip off to sleep on schedule Sunday night and awaken bright eyed Monday morning ready for work or play. I recommend a 6-milligram time-release formulation. Try this trick when crossing time zones, too, taking the melatonin an hour before bedtime at your new destination.

HAVE AN AGELESS DAY
Sleep

What you do all day can affect your nightly sleep. Keep these tips in mind so you can spend the night revitalizing with deep, long, healthy sleep.

- **Get up** at your regular time, 7 to 9 hours after you fell asleep.
- **Get out** into the bright daylight to set your circadian rhythms for restful sleep.
- **Work out** vigorously, the earlier in the day the better.
- **Challenge your mind** with mental activities such as reading, writing, socializing, games, analyses, and puzzles.
- **Relax or meditate** to relieve stress.
- **Seek help** for dysphoria or depression if you often feel sad or hopeless.
- **Stop stimulants** such as coffee or chocolate at your own cut-off time.
- **Unwind** in the final hour or so before bedtime. Turn off the television, turn on some soft music, dim the lights, soak in a hot bath, use relaxation or meditation techniques, and steer clear of tomorrow's to-do list.
- **Get to bed on time.** If you've followed the preceding steps, you should feel delightfully drowsy. Sweet dreams.

---

turing process, tryptophan supplements never returned to market. You can get a safe dose of tryptophan from warm milk or turkey, which helps to explain all those glazed looks after Thanksgiving dinner.

Medications That Interfere with Sleep

A number of over-the-counter and prescription medications can get in the way of a good night's sleep. Some to watch out for include certain decongestants (such as pseudoephedrine), beta blockers (such as Inderal), corticosteroids (such as hydrocortisone, prednisolone), some antidepressants (Prozac, Paxil, and Zoloft), thyroid hormones (such as Synthroid), antiepileptics (such as Dilantin), and bronchodilators (Isuprel).

If you're experiencing this very common side effect, report it to your doctor, who may guide you to trying alternative drugs, different dosages, or timing adjustments until the problem is eliminated.

Many life events can affect how you sleep—a new job, a move, a relationship's beginning or end, children, health conditions, even the seasons. Combined with the changes time brings to your body and brain, these variables can substantially affect the quality of your sleep, so don't rest on your laurels. Return to your sleep journal after any life shift that might affect your shut-eye; if you're feeling irritable, sleepy, or depressed; or simply to check in with yourself now and again. Remain conscious of your unconscious time to keep your Longevity Quotient high.

YOUR AGELESS AGENDA
Sleep and Relaxation

Check off each item as you achieve it:

☐ Seven to 9 hours of high-quality sleep every night that leaves you alert and refreshed through the following day
☐ Daily exercise for 30 minutes or more
☐ Daily bright light exposure for 30 minutes or more
☐ A dark, quiet sleeping environment
☐ Ability to relax before sleep and after nighttime awakenings
☐ Good sleep habits
☐ Freedom from sleep medications

CHAPTER 6

ENGAGEMENT

OLD ENGAGEMENT RULE	NEW ENGAGEMENT RULE
Avoid stress.	**#1.** Respond successfully to stress.
Prepare for the worst.	**#2.** Expect the best.
Put career first.	**#3.** Put relationships first.
Retire and leave all your cares behind.	**#4.** Stay active and engaged.
Leave sex for the young and beautiful.	**#5.** Stay sexually active.

A FRIEND OF MINE introduced me to the great comedian George Burns. We met at the Hillcrest Country Club in Los Angeles where Burns came every day to play bridge. Burns had a great attitude toward life. Age 96 at that time, he told me that the secret to his longevity was pretty simple. He didn't eat too much, since no one paid him to eat; he exercised every day; and sex was fine "as long as you don't inhale." (He emphasized this last point by taking a puff from his famous stogie.) The real key, though, said Burns, was that he couldn't die as long as he had a booking.

Burns understood the health-enhancing power of staying involved with life. During his eighties and nineties, he starred in two hit movies playing God (talk about making the connection!), recorded a country and western album, and wrote a best-selling book, *How to Live to Be 100 or More*—dedicated to the widows of his last six physicians. George made it to his goal: He was performing right up to his death at age 100.

WHAT'S YOUR LONGEVITY QUOTIENT?

Engagement

To assess your longevity quotient in social and psychological habits, take the following quiz. Answer each of the questions with a rating on a scale of 0 to 10, using the suggested descriptions of the scale as a guide. Enter the points in the "Your LQ Points" column. Be sure not to exceed the maximum score allowed for each item.

	Your LQ Points	Max LQ Points
How would you rate your emotional health?		
10 points: Great; I feel happy and enjoy my life pretty much all of the time		
0 points: I feel seriously depressed and/or unhappy most of the time	____	**10**
How would you rate your optimism?		
10 points: I always expect the best, even if I've just been disappointed		
0 points: I always expect the worst so I'm never disappointed	____	**10**
How successful do you feel you are at coping with stress?		
10 points: I can handle whatever comes my way by relying on responses and stress management techniques that I've found to work for me		
0 points: Stress upsets me so much that I do my best to avoid it	____	**10**
How happy are you about your social and family connections?		
10 points: I feel supported by and supportive of wonderful people whom I'm happy to have in my life		
0 points: I'm quite unhappy about the state of my family and/or social life	____	**10**
In an emergency, how many people could you rely on to help you in some way? Score 2 points for each person up to a total of 10 points.		
10 points: 5 or more people		
0 points: no one	____	**10**

	Your LQ Points	Max LQ Points

How's your sex life?

10 points: Great—satisfying and as active as I want it to be

10 points: I would like an active sex life but have no partner
at present

0 points: I'm not having sex because I've lost interest   _____   **10**

How would you rate your level of active participation in life?

10 points: I pursue my interests with passion and am always
open to new experiences

0 points: I try to minimize my exertion and stay within my   _____   **10**
comfort zone

Do you participate in volunteer work or service activities?

10 points: Yes, I make it a point to give to others on an
ongoing basis, and I enjoy doing so

0 points: No, I have no particular interest in volunteering   _____   **10**

**How would you rate your past experience and current
interest in education?**

10 points: High; learning new things is a top priority and
source of genuine pleasure

0 points: I prefer just to be entertained   _____   **10**

What's your level of financial comfort?

10 points: I am financially secure

0 points: I'm in financial distress without a plan for the present
or future   _____   **10**

Total   _____   **100**

What does your engagement LQ say about your psychological and social health? To see how your thoughts, feelings, and coping behaviors are contributing to your healthspan, check the Dean's diagnosis for your score.

Total LQ Score	The Dean's Diagnosis
91–100	You're making the connection to a long, happy life. Congratulations and keep it up.
81–90	You're well-engaged with life but may want to take a look at some of your low-scoring areas to optimize your health and happiness.

71–80   You're in danger of disconnecting. Your attitudes and behaviors could be limiting your potential and harming your health. Let the New Rules guide you to how you can improve.

61–70   Engagement emergency. Changing the way you engage with the world is vital to your LQ. Get started today.

60 or below   Rejoin the world! You need an overhaul of your social and psychological habits. You must make a change if you hope for an enjoyable, fulfilling lifespan.

The Toxic Effects of Stress

There's no doubt about it, stress ages us. Stress triggers our body's fight-or-flight response, originally designed to keep us out of harm's way in an era of charging mastodons and saber-toothed tigers. The stress response prepares us for peak performance in the moment of truth. When we sense danger, our brains signal our adrenal glands to release the stress hormones adrenaline and cortisol. These hormones trigger a flurry of reactions that include sending blood from our internal organs to our muscles to prepare us for action, boosting blood sugar to give us extra fuel, shutting off some immune system activity to conserve our energy, and raising our heart rates and blood pressures for that quick burst of effort to get us back to our caves alive. Like our prehistoric forebearers, we're programmed with all the physiological responses necessary for surviving life-threatening danger.

AGELESS REWARDS
Engagement

A healthy mind-set and coping style can make your life longer and better by:

- Protecting against heart disease and stroke
- Improving immunity
- Preventing memory loss and keeping your mind sharp
- Reducing the risk of ulcers and colitis
- Improving sleep
- Establishing support networks to help you surmount life's challenges
- Maintaining physical mobility and skills

Fast-forward to the third millennium. You live in the suburbs, and instead of saber-toothed tigers you have countless small stresses to deal with each day—traffic, deadlines, getting your kids to do their homework, jury duty, handling an unenlightened boss or slow employees, disagreements with your spouse, caring for aging parents. Such challenges are rarely conquered by a quick burst of energy. They're built in to life—and if each one triggers the stress response, the effect can be toxic.

NEW ENGAGEMENT RULE #1:
RESPOND SUCCESSFULLY TO STRESS

The occasional shower of adrenal hormones that enabled our ancestors to survive predators' attacks probably didn't produce lasting problems in their short lives. However, the long-term exposure to high levels of stress hormones characteristic of modern living may contribute to a host of life-threatening chronic diseases—hypertension, heart disease and stroke, ulcers, and colitis. Stress hormones raise blood pressure, elevate adrenal steroid levels, and increase production of an inflammatory protein called interleukin-6, which dampens immune responses and can lead to hyperimmune diseases. Stress hormones can also flood your digestive system with acid.

In addition to producing stress hormones, negative emotions can stimulate production of substances called proinflammatory cytokines, which attack the immune system and may contribute to or affect the course of diseases such as heart disease, osteoporosis, arthritis, type 2 diabetes, and memory loss. These inflammatory agents can also impede wound healing and recovery from infection.

Stress also has a toxic effect on the brain. Among the chemicals released by stress are catecholamines, which interfere with key brain cell receptors and the supply of glucose that fuels brain function. Another class of stress-related brain chemicals is glucocorticoids, which limit synaptic plasticity—the degree to which brain cells can communicate—over the course of hours, and can impact dendrite structure (branchlike connectors between brain cells) for weeks. Prolonged stress exposure can cause loss of brain cells, particularly in the hippocampus, an important memory center.

Stress Better (Not Necessarily Less)

You've heard the mantra: Stress less! You hear it so often it probably just adds to the pressure as your emotional mercury starts to rise. For most people, the advice to stress less is not just impossible but wrong. A certain amount of stress comes with living a rich, loving, rewarding, involved life. It's not how much stress you have but how you handle it that matters most for your health.

When I was writing this book, my wife was spending 3 or 4 days a week in Berkeley, California, 400 miles from our home in Los Angeles, taking courses in art history at the Graduate Theological Seminary and the University of California. This means that while Leah immersed herself in the great artwork of the 15th century, I was a full-time dean, full-time book author, and full-time dad. I had to do a lot of juggling and role changing to pull it all off. I also made darn sure to exercise regularly, eat right, get enough sleep, and laugh as much as I can, because without these coping mechanisms, these pressures could quickly turn into unhealthy stress.

So it was that I was in the middle of a set of tennis the other day when I got a call on my cell phone. It was my 9-year-old son, Isaac. He had some bad news. The housekeeper had run over his cello.

As you may know, a cello is a large but delicate wooden instrument worth a good deal of money. It's not meant for encounters with car wheels. I could have reacted to this mishap in a number of ways. Let's see; I could have yelled at Isaac for leaving his cello in the driveway; chastised the housekeeper for backing over the thing; become angry with my wife for being in Berkeley, far away from the mess; or gotten mad at myself for being on the tennis court instead of at home keeping an eye on things.

Instead, I told Isaac that I was glad it was his cello that got hit and not him. (I did emphasize that this type of accident should be a once in a lifetime event.) Then I stepped up my tennis game and used the residual adrenaline in my bloodstream to win the set.

These things happen all the time. Can you or I prevent them? In retrospect I could have given my son piano lessons, since pianos are much

React and Get Plaque

The Kuopio Ischemic Heart Disease Study put 901 Finnish men aged 42 to 60 under mental stress, measured how much their blood pressure leaped, then looked at the plaque in their arteries. The researchers found that the men whose blood pressures rose most in response to stress had the most arterial plaque, a symptom of heart disease.

Successful versus Nonsuccessful Ways to Cope with Stress

In his book *Aging Well*, Dr. George Vaillant describes adaptive and maladaptive coping techniques that people use when faced with stress. To follow New Rule #1, choose from the "Successful" column—sublimation, humor, altruism, suppression, and perspective.

Unsuccessful	Successful
Projection: Attribute the problem to others.	**Sublimation:** Turn bad situations into good.
Passive aggression: Channel your anger into this unproductive activity.	**Humor:** Laugh at yourself and the situation.
Dissociation: Hey, it's not your problem.	**Altruism:** Get pleasure from helping others in similar situations.
Acting out: Respond like a child.	**Suppression** (not repression): Be patient and look for the bright side.
Fantasy: Get me to Shangri-la!	**Perspective:** Put the situation in its proper place.

Adapted from *Aging Well*, George Vaillant, Little, Brown and Company, Boston, 2002.

less likely to get run over, or sent him to military school where the instruments are made of brass instead of wood. I could have had my housekeeper walk my kids the 2½ miles to school. But only hindsight is 20/20. We can't stop most of the fender benders of life from happening, nor should we spend our lives trying. However, we *can* resond effectively to the stress response with New Rules techniques.

Managing Anger

Anger kills—and not just when someone stuck in freeway traffic takes out a gun and starts shooting. Studies have linked long-term patterns of anger, hostility, and frustration to substantial increases in heart attack risk, as high as threefold or more. In addition to being hard on relationships and your emotional health, anger can also trigger the stress response to accelerate aging in your body.

One study assessed the anger response levels of 1,305 older men without heart disease, then followed them for 7 years to track instances of heart attack. During this time, the men with the highest anger levels were three times more likely to have a heart attack than the least angry participants. Another study of 13,000 men and women aged 45 to 64 had similar results. Using a 10-point anger scale, researchers found that those who are highly prone to anger have nearly triple the risk of heart attack. About 8 percent of participants were in this high-risk range.

Anger may start to attack your health quite young, suggests a study that assessed the hostility levels of 374 men and women aged 18 to 30, then used electron beam tomography to measure calcifications in their arteries. The researchers repeated the hostility assessment and tomography test 5 and 10 years later. Participants with above-average hostility ratings had 2.5 times more risk of arterial calcifications, early signs of cardiovascular disease.

Are you doomed if you're naturally quick on the draw? Not if you learn to manage your anger. Anger management strategies can help stop the spiral of feelings and hormones that leads to hostility, frustration, and rage. Studies have also shown that learning to reduce and manage emotional distress can improve your chances of surviving a heart attack.

Personally, I don't like driving, but I spend plenty of time on the road driving to work and the kids to school, ball games, play dates, and music lessons. How do I cope with the congested Los Angeles traffic without getting hot under the collar? I pop the latest John Grisham novel or a new biography into the tape deck and listen. The time flies so fast that the next thing I know I'm sitting in the car in my garage, listening until the end of the chapter.

Everyone has favorite coping mechanisms. The first step is to figure out what's really making you mad. Is it the traffic or is thinking about someone at work making you tense? Track the triggers for anger in your daily life. Get conscious of what you are feeling. The more aware you become of your sensations, emotions, and thoughts, the farther outside the feeling you can stand, gradually seeing the situation more clearly—and objectively. Next, consciously respond. Look for solutions. You may need to renegotiate how to discuss household finances with your partner, or air a grievance to the appropriate person at work, or reevaluate your own response. Do you have to get mad every time someone cuts you off, or can you make up a funny nickname for their car instead?

Other effective anger diffusing techniques are meditation, progressive relaxation, deep breathing, and exercise. You may find that one works better for you.

Finally, practicing AgeLess rules for sleep, exercise, and nutrition will physically prepare your body to better handle anger and stress. And you may find that caring for yourself makes you less likely to get mad at the world.

Relax and Meditate: The Zen of Longevity

Meditation and progressive relaxation are great antidotes to stress. The body slows down to a sleeplike pace, but the mind remains in the relaxed-alert alpha wave range. Learning to relax or meditate can be a great boost to your healthspan, so invest the time now and turn to these techniques whenever you need them. Try to establish a regular schedule—perhaps first thing in the morning or the last thing you do before going to bed at night.

Here's one simple form of meditation to try. Like most skills, meditation gets better with practice, so don't give up if you don't feel particularly meditative your first time.

- Begin your session by sitting or lying in a comfortable position, close your eyes, and breathe easily through your nose. It's recommended that you wait for at least 2 hours after eating a meal before meditating.
- Focus your attention on each muscle group in your body, starting with your feet and working your way up to your face and head. Tense the muscles you're working with, then let them go. Take a deep breath in and out, letting your muscles relax completely. Move on to the next group.
- When you've relaxed all the muscles in your body, shift your focus to your breathing. Silently say your favorite calming word with each inhalation and exhalation. If you don't have a favorite word, say "AgeLess" with each breath.
- If thoughts come into your mind, gently set them aside and redirect your attention to your word.
- Continue for 10 to 20 minutes, or longer if you like.

Relaxation for Smokers

⑥ Whenever you want to light up in a moment of stress, meditate instead. You'll start to break the connection between stress and cigarettes.

⑥ If you're trying to quit, consider hypnosis therapy. Some people find it very effective, and it may help train your mind for meditation and sleep, too.

NEW ENGAGEMENT RULE #2:
EXPECT THE BEST

Is your glass half full or half empty? Do you see a happy, upbeat mood as an optional and occasional indulgence, to be expected only when falling in love, after the birth of a child, or upon getting a big promotion? As an unabashed optimist, I was very pleased when a study came out of the Mayo Clinic showing the power of positive thinking. Researchers interviewed 800 Minnesota residents to assess and rate their optimism levels, then tracked them for 35 years to see how long they lived. Regardless of age or sex, the optimists lived longer. The pessimists died prematurely. In fact, for every 10 percent increase in the pessimism index, there were 20 percent more early deaths.

Many other studies affirm that happy people are healthier and outsurvive their pessimistic or depressed counterparts—and the benefits of a good mood can obviously begin today. When the Veterans Administration Normative Aging Study took a longitudinal look at 659 men in middle and older age, researchers found that optimism was associated with feelings of better health, more vitality, higher mental health ratings, and lower levels of pain. Depression had the opposite effect. Feeling good is not a luxury; it's a basic component of health. Engaging the world with an expectation of the best can give you a longer, better life.

The High Cost of Depression

In the United States, 19 million people are affected by depression, and its toll in death and disability equals that of heart disease. In fact, one of the best predictors of how well you'll age is your depression level.

DR. ROBERT SAPOLSKY'S

Top 10 Tips for Dealing Effectively with Stress

Stanford biology professor and MacArthur Fellow Robert Sapolsky can keep you quite entertained with graphic descriptions of stress and the havoc it wreaks on your body and mind. Fortunately, the author of *Why Zebras Don't Get Ulcers* is a practical man who can also help you cope. Try Dr. Sapolsky's top 10 tips for dealing more effectively with stress:

1. **Don't try to control the uncontrollable.** Though a sense of control can help reduce certain sorts of stress, trying to exert your personal power over uncontrollable situations just sets you up to feel at fault.
2. **One step at a time.** In the face of a major, seemingly insurmountable stressor, the old cliché really can work wonders.
3. **Look down the pike and plan.** If you can't prevent a stressor from happening, at least get some predictive information about when it's coming, how bad it's going to be, and how long it will last. This helps you plan your coping strategy for the stressful time and lets you know when it's all over so you can finally relax.
4. **Check your age, then change or accommodate.** In general, younger people prefer to reduce stress by changing the stressor, while older people are likely to find relief in accommodating the stressor instead.
5. **Choose your own best coping technique.** Just because a stress management technique works for a friend doesn't mean it will for you. One person's

When it leads to self-destructive, high-risk behaviors such as attempting suicide, depression can be a literal death sentence. Depression also increases your risk of heart disease, stroke, osteoporosis, and hyperimmune and gastrointestinal diseases.

Being depressed increases your risk of heart disease by an astonishing 40 percent and can also make a fatal heart attack more likely if you already have heart disease. Sometimes receiving a diagnosis of heart disease or a first heart attack can exacerbate existing depression or may lead to depression's onset, causing a potentially deadly downward spiral.

Several factors make depression hard on your heart. The stress hormones triggered by depression can accelerate arteriosclerosis (hardening of the arteries) and raise blood pressure. Catecholamines, a stress reducer is the next person's stressor. Listen to advice, try new techniques, but choose what works best for you.

6. **Don't fall for stress pseudoscience.** Despite what some might say, no brand of stress management has been scientifically proven to work better than the rest. It's true that various interventions—meditation, prayer, aerobic exercise, hobbies, relaxation therapy—have been found to be effective for different people, but again, what matters is managing *your* stress well.

7. **Don't save your stress management for the weekend** or for the 15 seconds when you're on hold on the phone. Set aside time to practice your stress management techniques on an almost daily basis.

8. **Don't avoid getting ulcers by giving them to everyone around you.** Unfortunately, some people choose to reduce stress by taking it out on someone else. Not only is this hard on your social networks, but you're likely to feel guilty, which makes you even more stressed than before you handed off the torch.

9. **Do unto others.** If you feel like you're drowning in your own stress and problems, find a way to help someone else.

10. **Reach out.** The world's most powerful stress reducer is probably a shoulder to cry on. For social primates such as us, isolation is an aching stressor and a major risk factor for our health.

Get the full scoop on stress and how you can control your own response in Dr. Sapolsky's book *Why Zebras Don't Get Ulcers: An Updated Guide to Stress, Stress-Related Diseases, and Coping* (WH Freeman & Co.).

particular class of stress hormone secreted at higher levels by people who are depressed, can cause abnormal heart rhythms, which may be fatal. Depression can also lead to increased production of C-reactive protein (CRP), which is a substantial risk factor for heart disease. People with heart disease who suffer from depression have a higher mortality rate independent of the severity of their disease.

Depression Kills

A 6-year study published in 2000 found that people with high depressive symptoms at the study's start had a 24 percent higher risk of dying from all causes.

Researchers at Duke University assessed the depression levels of 1,250 people with heart disease, then followed them for 19 years. Depressed patients had substantially higher risks of dying from heart and other diseases. Patients who were moderately to severely depressed at the study's start were 69 percent more likely to die of heart disease over the course of the study. People with mild depression had a less dramatic but still significant 20 to 30 percent increase in risk of death over all the study's time frames.

Your risk of stroke also goes up dramatically if you are depressed. A study of 6,676 adults in Alameda County in California followed participants for 29 years. Those people with five or more depressive symptoms when the study started were 54 percent more likely to have a stroke in the next three decades than those without depressive symptoms. Another study found that middle-age men who suffered from depression and anxiety were three times more likely to have a stroke than men who weren't depressed.

Feeling bad can even penetrate to your bones. Depression increases the production of corticosteroids, steroidlike chemicals that can reduce bone density. Feeling depressed is also likely to cause you to skip exercise and miss your calcium dose, both important to bone strength.

Depression and Age

As we age, we are more likely to experience life events that precipitate depression. Your chances of losing a loved one increase. Your children leave home. You may not have achieved your highest career goals. Perhaps your life didn't follow the script you wrote for it when you were young, or you don't have the nest egg you think you need. Women face the additional challenge of menopause, when depression is a common symptom.

The good news is that though feeling some depression as you age may be likely, there's a lot you can do to prevent and treat it. Today's aging generation faces more options than ever before for safeguarding emotional health through the golden years. Most depressed individuals respond to a combination of short-term psychotherapy and medication. As the severity and type of depression can vary widely from one person to the next, treatment can be tailored to individual needs. Two types of short-term therapy are often successful in treat-

Depression Checklist

According to the National Institute of Mental Health, you are considered clinically depressed if you've felt sad, low, and without energy for 2 weeks or more and you have five or more of the following symptoms:

☐ Persistent sad, anxious, or empty mood
☐ Feelings of hopelessness or pessimism
☐ Feelings of guilt, worthlessness, or helplessness
☐ Loss of interest or pleasure in activities you once enjoyed, including sex
☐ Decreased energy, fatigue, or feeling slowed down
☐ Difficulty concentrating, remembering, or making decisions
☐ Insomnia, early morning awakening, or oversleeping
☐ Appetite loss and/or weight loss or overeating and/or weight gain
☐ Thoughts of death or suicide; suicide attempts
☐ Restlessness; irritability
☐ Persistent physical symptoms that don't respond to treatment, such as headaches, digestive disorders, or chronic pain

If you meet the criteria for depression, talk to your doctor today.

ing depression: interpersonal and cognitive/behavioral therapies. Interpersonal therapy examines the relationships that may have led to depression and continue to feed depressed feelings. Cognitive/behavioral therapy, by contrast, identifies individual behaviors and thought patterns that perpetuate depression and helps the patient to change them.

The list of drugs successfully deployed to treat depression has grown dramatically over the past few decades, enabling doctors and patients to find the medication that balances the greatest therapeutic effect with the fewest side effects. Many of the top sellers work by increasing levels of the brain chemical serotonin; these selective serotonin reuptake inhibitors (SSRIs) include Prozac, Paxil, and Zoloft. Wellbutrin is another new effective antidepressant, though its mechanism of action is still unknown.

There are also lifestyle measures that can help prevent or alleviate depression. Aerobic exercise and weight training are wonderful anti-

St. John's Wort

St. John's wort is extensively used in Europe and the United States to treat mild to moderate depression. But we still don't know its effectiveness for more serious depression. Some clinical trials have shown positive results for mild to moderate depression while others find no effect for moderate to severe depression.

Because herbal supplements are relatively unregulated in this country, one of the biggest concerns with St. John's wort is knowing what's in your pills. It may not be what the bottle says. The *Los Angeles Times* obtained bottles of St. John's wort from 10 different manufacturers and sent them to an independent laboratory for testing. The lab found that the quantity of the actual active ingredient in the pills ranged from 30 percent to 140 percent of the amount indicated on the label. When the makers complained that the lab didn't perform the test right, the *L.A. Times* sent the bottles to a second lab and confirmed the first lab's measurements.

This variability in active ingredient levels prevents most doctors from prescribing St. John's wort for mild depression, as is commonly done in Europe. If you choose to take St. John's wort, stick with the same brand in the hope that the next batch will be the same strength as the last one. Always tell your doctor about all medications you're taking, including herbs.

dotes for depression. Loneliness is a major cause of depression among seniors, and having friends or family members to confide in can make a real difference. Volunteering to help others is another way to feel happier yourself. A Canadian study of 887 depressed patients with heart disease found that three factors helped to improve survival rates: the individual's perception of having enough social support; regular contact (monthly or more often), in person or on the phone, with friends and relatives; and living with another person.

NEW ENGAGEMENT RULE #3:
PUT RELATIONSHIPS FIRST

How well you age is deeply dependent upon your relationships with others. From how much respect and autonomy you get in your current job to how easily you turn to friends for stress-relieving support, whether you have a partner to stand by you as the challenges of old age mount, and how highly you think of yourself, the people in your life affect its quality and quantity in very discernible ways.

Social Networks Can Save Your Life

Psychologists and sociologists use the technical term *social networks* to describe what you may more commonly think of as the people in your life: family; friends; work buddies; and people you know from church, sports, volunteer work, hobby groups, or school. Those people can help you manage stress, boost your morale and self-esteem, and enhance your satisfaction with life—all of which improve your longevity prospects. If you get sick or hurt, have a financial crash, or face an emotional crisis, your social network can help to care for you and offer ideas and resources to get you through. Having social connections has also been found to improve people's access to health and social services.

Women are generally better at building and maintaining social networks than men. When men gather on the basketball court or football field, they are usually more intent on beating their opponents than getting to know them well. Women, on the other hand, often do the lion's share of running the family, managing the social calendar, talking on the phone with friends, going to lunch with coworkers, volunteering, and joining clubs. These sorts of uncompetitive personal connections tend to weave a wider, stronger net. Many single guys know the double whammy of breaking up a relationship—you lose most of your friends along with your girlfriend or wife, which can be one of the reasons that widowers tend to die much sooner after losing their wives than do widows after the loss of their husbands.

Socializing Keeps You Spry

The MacArthur Foundation Study of Successful Aging selected a group of high-functioning men and women ages 70 to 79 and followed them for 7 years. Over the study period, the participants with more social ties showed better maintenance of their daily activities.

Diversify

When it comes to social connections, you don't want to put all your eggs in one basket. A study of 3,240 older North Carolinians found that social support generally helped to protect against physical decline, but the participants with more diverse networks had higher morale than those who relied solely on family or an otherwise restricted group.

Your Significant Other Provides Support

We've known for some time that being happily married improves your health and increases your lifespan. A spouse provides the closest form of life-extending social support, keeping you well with companionship and love—both primal human needs—and help with practical tasks. If you develop health problems, your partner may serve as the chief caregiver, assisting in daily activities, serving meals, and providing nursing care; coordinating medical treatment with your doctors; researching options and alternatives; and keeping you company.

While both sexes benefit from marriage, men seem to get the biggest healthspan boost from tying the knot. This may be because women are more adept at maintaining outside social networks to sustain them in the absence of a partner, tend to care more closely for their own health, and are more resilient.

Though most of the research on partnership and longevity has looked at traditional married couples, stable long-term relationships outside of marriage have similar effects. It's also clear that dysfunctional and abusive marriages can negatively impact healthspan. Your investment in a *healthy, mutually supportive* partnership may be the best one you ever make for your long, happy life.

Self-Esteem Helps, Too

Once you've got your social network in place, you might want to start working on your self-esteem. Imagine everybody's dream come true: You've been nominated for an Academy Award. A billion people are watching around the world. You're wearing couture and jewels that you didn't even have to pay for and smiling for the cameras. You're a certified star—but in your category, only one can win and guess what? The star who walks away with the Oscar will, on average, live 3.6 years longer than those who were nominated but did not win—this is an impressive and very significant increase in life expectancy.

This surprising finding is not Hollywood hype but a well-researched study of all the Oscar nominees for best lead and supporting actor and actress since the awards' inception—a total of 1,649 people. After controlling for other variables, researchers found that the winning performers enjoyed this 3.6-year longevity edge over the other nominees and lived 3.9 years longer than their fellow actors appearing in the same films. What's fascinating about this result is that while many studies have found that people with higher social status have longer lives, it was widely believed that the poor nutrition and housing, higher stress, and lack of health care associated with lower-paying jobs shortened the lifespans of people on the low end of the social scale. However, Oscar nominees who lose don't face any of these problems. These winners appear to live longer purely through higher self-esteem.

Widowers Die Prematurely

Losing a wife is one of the worst things that can happen to a man's longevity. Leonard Davis was a great visionary. He was a pioneer in providing car, health and life insurance to seniors at a time when others refused to enroll them. With Ethel Percy Andrus, he cofounded AARP, and his administrative talents helped this organization grow rapidly. He chose the site for the memorial to Ethel Percy Andrus here at USC. Then, he endowed the first School of Gerontology, where I have the honor of being the dean. He knew a lot about successful aging, but when his wife Sophie died, Leonard became deeply depressed and seemed to care little about life. Despite the best medical care and the support of his children and friends, Leonard lasted only a few months past Sophie.

Even successful, strong-willed men like Leonard Davis have a hard time surviving after their wives die. Developing your social network can help you face such a loss and regain your will to live.

Most of us can't count on winning an Oscar as a longevity-boosting technique, but good self-esteem and self-efficacy (belief in one's ability to organize and execute actions to achieve specific goals) are two traits that can help you live a long, rewarding life. Following the New Rules in this chapter can help nurture self-esteem and self-efficacy. Find effective ways to respond to stress, foster an optimistic outlook, invest in a good marriage or partnership and strong social support network, take on challenges and see them through, volunteer in community activities, and, if you have a partner, enjoy a healthy sex life.

Religion Can Enhance Healthspan

Another relationship that can enhance your healthspan is a spiritual one. A number of studies have shown that people who regularly attend religious services live longer and have fewer illnesses than the less devout. The classic study that uncovered this connection followed 3,968 individuals, ages 65 to 101, for 6 years. It showed that just believing wasn't enough. Those who attended services at least once a week had a 46 percent increase in life expectancy when compared with other study participants. In contrast, people who stuck to private prayer, Bible reading, and religious television or radio were more likely to have poor health. This wasn't due to health problems at the beginning of the study that kept these participants at home, since the researchers took this into account.

Attending religious services may improve healthspan by reducing depression, promoting stability in marriage, lending support in times of illness and disability, and offering a meaning for life—a reason to cope and survive. Participating in a spiritual community can provide salvation right here on earth.

Believe in Yourself
for a Better Healthspan

The MacArthur Foundation Study of Successful Aging found that individuals who scored high on measures of self-efficacy did very well in their old age. Believing in yourself is a great longevity aid.

Improve Your Healthspan with Religion

A Duke University study of 4,000 people ages 65 and older found that those who attend religious services regularly:

- Have 50 percent less depression
- Have lower blood pressure
- Are less likely to smoke or be alcoholics

NEW ENGAGEMENT RULE #4:
STAY ACTIVE AND ENGAGED

Staying active and involved with life—whether through volunteer work, study, an artistic pursuit, or travel—is also important to your healthspan. Take the case of Margaret and John, both in their seventies and suffering from the same sort of crippling arthritis. While John sits in his recliner watching old movies and game shows on television and complains bitterly about his misfortune, Margaret takes classes at the senior center, does aqua aerobics at the local pool, and looks forward to acting in an upcoming musical comedy. Guess who's likely to get sick and die first?

Staying physically and mentally active sends healthy messages to the body and brain. Being involved also helps with New Rules #1 to #3 by helping to beat stress, boost mood, and keep social relationships strong.

Brainpower: Stay Active to Build It

Just as aerobic exercise and weight training build bone and muscle strength, mental exercise can build brainpower. The more you engage in mentally challenging activities, the better your chances for preserving brain function as you age. Professional development, taking or teaching classes, joining a book club, and even working crossword puzzles are all ways to keep your brain healthy and your mind quick. In fact, one of the consistent findings in aging research is that people with the most education have the least risk of Alzheimer's and other diseases.

Evidence indicates that actively using your mind can spur neurogenesis, or the production of new brain cells, as well as arborization—the forming of connections between them. This additional brain reserve

Your Brain: Use It or Lose It

In a study of 2,000 older French men and women, those who actively participated in social or leisure activities such as traveling, gardening, or knitting had a significantly lower risk of Alzheimer's disease.

may make the difference between getting Alzheimer's disease or not, as well as keeping day-to-day memory and mental function sharp.

Retirement: Don't Let It Be Toxic

In a Fort Lauderdale supermarket, I found my groceries being packed by an older man with a merry smile. He insisted on carrying them to the car and loading them into the trunk. My bagman was a former advertising executive who retired to Florida at age 65 expecting to play golf, take it easy, and reap the rewards of years of hard work. Two years later, bored, depressed, and yearning to be around people again, he took the supermarket job not because he needed money, but because he liked the sense of purpose and social connection it gave him. And the exercise kept him trim. You could call this man a recovering retiree.

Up until the 20th century, retirement was a luxury available to a few very wealthy individuals. Most old folks lived with their children, worked as long as they could, and relied on their families for support and care. With the introduction in the 20th century of Social Security, Medicare, and pension plans, the shape of later years has dramatically changed. Millions of Americans have "retired"—stopped working to take an extended vacation, which many people view as their ultimate reward.

The average age of retirement has declined over the past few decades. Many people are closing up shop in their early sixties or even late fifties, lured by early-retirement incentive packages and the prospect of escaping the rat race. This trend has combined with increased lifespan to create retirements so long they may even surpass the time spent working.

Some individuals thrive in retirement, staying active and realizing long-held dreams—spending more time with grandchildren, learning to paint, writing a novel, traveling the world. For others, retirement can be a disappointment, even toxic. The loss of identity, purpose, and self-worth associated with stopping work can rapidly lead to depression. When not well-planned, retirement can be a passport to disability and death.

Work challenges us mentally, connects us to people, and gives us a sense of structure, purpose, and worth. One solution is to simply not retire. The writer, Mildred Benson, author of the original Nancy Drew mysteries, recently died at the ripe old age of 96. Mildred spent 58 years as a journalist and wrote more than 130 books. The day of her death found her at her desk at the newspaper *The Blade*, where she wrote a weekly column. She had suffered from lung cancer for the past 5 years but never stopped working. Mildred fell ill at the office, went to the hospital, and was gone by the end of the day.

Exercise Your Brain

Here are some ideas for boosting your brainpower through mental exercise:

- Professional education opportunities in your field (conferences, seminars, in-service days)
- A new job; maybe even a new career
- Extension classes at local colleges
- Internet courses
- Book clubs
- Research and writing—sign up to be the researcher or write the newsletter for a group or cause you're involved with
- Hobbies
- Lectures at bookstores, libraries, museums, and other venues
- Alumni programs offered by your alma mater
- Teaching what you know—through youth groups, professional or volunteer organizations, grass-roots gatherings, or local colleges and extension programs
- Elderhostel, where you can spend a week learning new subjects at colleges and universities across the nation
- Living in one of the active retirement communities linked to a university campus, with easy access to ongoing education

Another AgeLess tactic is to make the transition to a healthy, engaging, and activity-filled retirement by planning ahead. Start by making three lists of things you plan to, hope to, and dream of doing in retirement. Try out some of these activities in advance of retirement day. Take a cruise, spend a week with your grandchildren, start your novel. Are they as pleasurable and meaningful as you had hoped? Do they provide enough social interaction to keep you connected? Adjust your lists accordingly.

Plan your retirement finances carefully. It's hard to stay positive when you have to watch every dollar you spend or worry that your bank balance will expire before you do. Many financial advisors specialize in retirement planning and can help you with special issues such as retirement fund withdrawals, health care, estate planning, and insurance.

NEW ENGAGEMENT RULE #5:
STAY SEXUALLY ACTIVE

A sexy attitude is great for your healthspan—and it doesn't have to fade with age. Though most middle-age couples would be more shocked to find their parents being intimate in the upstairs bedroom than their teenager having sex in the basement, sex does not stop with the first gray hair! If you adopt an AgeLess lifestyle, there's no reason you can't enjoy a robust sex life into your eighties and beyond.

A healthy sex life can help you age well on many fronts. First, you get physical exercise. The average American couple takes 10 to 16 minutes for sex, which counts as a full exercise bout. Of course, longer time can be enjoyably taken and more exercise obtained. Sex can also boost your mood, offering a natural high that draws on your full neuroendocrine response to send feel-good messages to the brain. And as the ultimate act of intimacy, sex is a wonderful way to nurture your connection to

Safe Sex Is the New Rule

Whatever your age, it's critical for your healthspan that you practice safe sex with any new partner.

What Do Seniors Look For in a Sexual Partner?

A study by the National Council on Aging asked what people with a lifetime of experience behind them looked for in a sexual partner. Men and women alike want someone with:

- High moral character
- Pleasant personality
- Good sense of humor
- Intelligence

Women in particular sought:

- Financial security
- Compatible religion

Men in particular sought (some things never change):

- Someone who likes sex
- Attractive body shape

your significant other. This loving bond not only gives life meaning but improves health and longevity, too.

Sex and Aging

I've been an advisor to two large studies on sexuality and aging, one by the AARP and another by the National Council on Aging (NCOA). The results from both studies were reassuring: The majority of seniors are sexually active and pleased with the quality and quantity of their love lives.

For most people, sex changes with age: We slow down physically; it takes longer than it once did to get aroused, to achieve orgasm, and to get aroused again. Think of the tortoise and the hare, and take your time! If you follow the New Rules, you should have plenty to spend. And, of course, eating right and exercising regularly can help keep all systems go. (See chapters 2 and 3 for more on diet and fitness.) But even more importantly, research shows that even as physical stamina wanes, sex can

A Note to Women

Sexual turn-ons can come from many different stimuli—not just touch but also sight, smell, and feelings. Some evidence suggests that older men may need more visual stimulus than younger men do to get aroused, so don't neglect the lingerie just because you're past a certain age.

remain richly satisfying as it becomes less physical and more of an expression of intimacy and a relationship's deeper meaning. This is especially true if you've been with your partner for a long time.

Sex and the Older Woman

The good news is that the intensity, quality, and quantity of female orgasms do not decline with age. The bad news is that the arrival of menopause can dampen desire and make sex uncomfortable. Decreased libido can also come from depression, which is common with menopause or relationship problems. Seeking professional help for these concerns can help you weather this transition, preserving your healthy sex life and strengthening your emotional connection with your partner.

As for discomfort, the decline in estrogen levels with menopause can make the vaginal lining thinner and dryer, which for many women means that intercourse is painful. This situation can be effectively treated with topical estrogen preparations that restore vaginal linings without the systemic risk factors of taking estrogen orally (see chapter 7 on hormone replacement therapy). Options include creams, a vaginal ring inserted every 3 months (Estring), and vaginal tablets inserted daily for 2 weeks and weekly after that (Vagifem). Water-based lubricants (Astroglide, K-Y Jelly) can also prevent discomfort during sexual contact. Cotton underwear allows airflow to sensitive areas, avoiding the irritation synthetics can cause. Finally, sexual activity helps to maintain vaginal lubrication. So stay active.

Sex and the Older Man

It used to be thought that the male erectile problems associated with aging were mostly psychological in origin, but now we know that they are primarily physical—and many of them can be treated. Certain things you once took for granted do change with age, and needless to say these developments can take a psychological toll, too. From your fifties on, men might experience a longer time to get an erection; smaller, less rigid erections; a briefer period of awareness before orgasm; and smaller, less forceful ejaculation. You may also find that you lose your erection faster after sex and require a longer time between orgasms, extending to hours and even days. Meanwhile your fertility declines, though it continues up into the nineties.

But don't worry: You're not alone, and normal aging definitely does not have to dull your sex life. Any man who knows women knows it's quality, not quantity, that makes for great sex.

The erection connection. Not being able to have an erection is every man's greatest bedroom fear. Failure to "get it up" does end up happening to a lot of us, eventually. Erectile dysfunction, defined as the inability to get and keep an erection sufficient for sexual relations, may affect as many as 30 million American men. Its frequency is hard to determine, since most men don't report it to anyone, but it does tend to increase with age. (I'm not talking about the occasional failure after a stressful day or having drunk too much alcohol.) One estimate is that 20 percent of men ages 50 to 59 suffer from the condition, with the number rising as high as 67 percent for men ages 70 and above.

It was once thought that the main causes of erectile dysfunction were mental or just a normal part of the aging process. It's now clear that most problems are related to medical conditions or drugs. One of the most common causes of erectile dysfunction is depression, which is a double whammy since the most popular drugs used to treat depression can also impede arousal. Other medical conditions that can contribute to erectile dysfunction include diabetes, peripheral vascular disease, and spinal cord disease. Drugs that can cause trouble getting and keeping an erection include antidepressants, particularly Prozac, Paxil, and Zoloft, but not Wellbutrin; hypertension medications; vasodilators; anticholinergic medications; narcotics; nicotine; and alcohol.

Viagra and more. When Pfizer introduced the new drug sildenafil, also known as Viagra, in 1998, it quickly became the fastest-selling medication in history. A statistic published in a leading medical journal at the time pegged over half of men ages 50 to 70 as suffering from erec-

---

Engagement

Here are some of the daily practices that can shape and support your AgeLess attitude.

- ⑥ **Get out of bed!** Oversleeping can be a sign of depression.
- ⑥ **Self-monitor.** Note your stress and anger levels, and identify and practice effective response techniques.
- ⑥ **Take a relaxation break** when you need to.
- ⑥ **Call a friend,** take someone to lunch, drop an e-mail to a family member, or profess your love to your partner.
- ⑥ **Laugh.** If the people around you don't do the trick, go to a funny movie or read a humorous book. Smile at someone you wouldn't otherwise smile at.
- ⑥ **Enjoy yourself.** Schedule something you love today and every day—cooking a delicious meal, playing with the kids, working on your favorite hobby, or taking a relaxing bath.
- ⑥ **Help out.** Do something to help another, either through formal volunteer work or a random act of kindness.
- ⑥ **Challenge your mind** with a class, a high-quality book, a puzzle or game, or practicing the piano.
- ⑥ **Share intimacy** with your significant other.

---

tile dysfunction, which adds up to a lot of pent-up demand. Before Viagra came along, treatment options for all these frustrated men and their partners were not very attractive.

The NCOA study on sex and aging was sponsored by a grant from Pfizer, the maker of Viagra, and in order to avoid any possible conflict of interest, the first draft of the survey didn't include a question on whether survey takers would consider using a Viagra-like drug. I convinced NCOA that seniors would consider the survey outdated without such a question. It was added, and the response to Viagra was positive from men and women alike. Proven to improve the maintenance of erections and with users also reporting more satisfying orgasms, Viagra offers a new lease on love life to many couples.

Viagra is available in doses of 25, 50, and 100 milligrams, but the usual dosage is 50 milligrams. It takes about 45 minutes to reach full effect, then lasts for 3 to 4 hours, which should give you plenty of time. Most people tolerate the drug well. Common side effects include flushing, indigestion, blue vision, and headache. Individuals taking nitroglycerin and some other medications should not take Viagra.

YOUR AGELESS AGENDA
Engagement

Check off each item as you achieve it:

- ☐ Effective response to stress
- ☐ Optimism and humor
- ☐ Prevention or treatment of depression
- ☐ Partnership, friendship, and love
- ☐ Satisfying sex life
- ☐ A strong social network
- ☐ Active involvement in life
- ☐ Volunteer or service work
- ☐ Sense of financial security

CHAPTER 7

HORMONE REPLACEMENT

OLD HORMONE RULE	NEW HORMONE RULE
Women: Start estrogen/progesterone replacement in perimenopause and continue indefinitely.	**#1.** Women: Don't take hormone replacement unless severe menopausal symptoms warrant it.
Women: Estrogen is the only way to protect against the risks and symptoms of menopause.	**#2.** Women: Consider estrogen alternatives, but wisely.
Men: Fight the low libido and muscle loss of aging with testosterone.	**#3.** Men: Don't take testosterone unless your doctor recommends it.
Both sexes: Experiment freely with "fountain of youth" hormone supplements.	**#4.** Both sexes: Just say "no" to human growth hormone (HGH), DHEA, androstenedione, and melatonin.

LATELY, MARIA HAS BEEN HAVING TROUBLE sleeping through the night. During the day, her mood is all over the map. She can't go into a meeting without fear of a hot flash. And, at 47, she has a lackluster love life. Maria is perimenopausal, and she has some important decisions to make. Maria had always figured that she'd go the hormone replacement therapy (HRT) route when the time came, but new revelations about the increased risk of breast and ovarian cancer associated with estrogen and progestin replacement have made her reconsider. What's a smart woman to do?

David recently celebrated his 65th birthday but is feeling less than jubilant. He sees flab where once he saw firm muscle. His energy level is low. His belly has grown. His sex drive seems to be slipping away. David's father would have simply accepted these changes and found a hobby. But an onslaught of advertisements in David's daily e-mail trumpets new options. Modern pharmacology can manufacture any hormone you like, and the supplement makers claim that their pills can restore youth. Should David take the bait?

I meet people like David and Maria all the time. They come up to me at lectures, often holding a bestseller touting the latest miracle cure for aging and wanting to know if it's true. Can you really restart your sex life with testosterone? Or stay forever young with DHEA?

Hormones represent a kind of new frontier in medicine, one about which most Americans have heard lots of conflicting health claims. We know so little and hope for so much. We've had success treating illnesses caused by hormone deficiency: Replacing insulin, for example, the hormone that type 1 diabetics lack, can effectively treat diabetes, and thyroid hormone effectively treats many thyroid diseases. But when it comes to combating age, it's much less clear that hormone replacement is effective or safe. Among the most complex and powerful chemicals in the body, hormones hold both promise and risk. Because of the many unsettled questions about hormonal supplementation, I can't assess your hormone LQ—but I can give you information that can help you understand the issues. In this emerging field, it's important to make cautious and knowledgeable choices.

Hormones: Restorers of Youth?

Hormones are biochemicals produced by certain organs to act on other organs and tissues in order to promote various body functions. The female hormones estrogen and progesterone, for instance, produced by the ovaries, regulate a woman's menstrual cycle and help the uterus and breasts prepare for pregnancy. HGH, made in the pituitary gland, triggers the growth of muscles, bones, and tissues. The workaday hormone insulin, secreted by the pancreas, sweeps glucose out of the bloodstream and into cells where it is converted into energy. Melatonin, made by the brain's tiny pineal gland, sends us off to sleep each night. The stress hormones cortisol and adrenaline are good friends in an acute crisis but turn into enemies if stress becomes a chronic condition. There's no doubt about it, hormones are powerful catalytic agents, so powerful that surging levels can cause 16-year-olds to become addicted to the thrashing sounds of Limp Bizkit while their wane can keep their 48-year-old mothers awake all night.

The production and secretion of most hormones decrease with age. At menopause, women experience a dramatic drop in estrogen levels and a host of unpleasant symptoms from night sweats and hot flashes to an increased risk of heart disease and osteoporosis. Most men experience a decrease in testosterone, the male sex hormone that spurs sex drive and preserves lean body mass, energy, and cognitive function, but it's far less marked (see page 215).

Secretions of HGH and DHEA decrease with age for both men and women. HGH spurs bone and tissue growth. Your peak secretion of 1,000 to 1,500 micrograms a day in pubescence gradually declines to as little as 50 micrograms a day in older age. Sleep problems, which become increasingly common with age, can also interfere with HGH secretion. DHEA is not actually a hormone but can be converted into estrogen-like and testosterone-like compounds. Claims for its benefits are highly inflated (see page 219). The fact is that we don't know DHEA's function, but we do know that it peaks between the ages of 25 and 35, then gradually declines to significantly lower amount, by age 60. In the case of melatonin, which is related to the light-dark cycle and may play an important role in sleep promotion, aging changes not the total amount of hormone produced, but the timing of its release into the bloodstream.

This leads to the million-dollar question: Can replacing these hormones as they decline forestall Father Time—and if so, at what cost or risk?

The answers are as complicated as hormones' effects on body systems. Think of these chemicals as your body's chief communicators and of the current state of medicine like technology during the early days of the Internet. We understand the power of hormones, but we don't yet know how to harness it for longevity and health during the aging process. Hormones work in extremely complex ways. Each secretion can cause a cascade of other hormones in a biochemical game of tag. The stakes of this game can be high. Replacing or supplementing hormones can upset the body's delicate balance, and our understanding is currently too limited to write prescriptions that work in perfect concert with this elaborate system.

For instance, there's no question that hormone replacement therapy relieves menopausal symptoms and helps preserve bone mass—but four decades after these benefits made hormone replacement therapy commonplace, many women felt blindsided when the news broke in 2002 that the Women's Health Initiative (WHI) study was stopped 3 years earlier than planned because the results clearly showed that the risks of taking estrogen and progestin outweighed their benefits. Findings of increased risks of heart attack, stroke, breast cancer, pulmonary embolism, and gallbladder disease lead the researchers to issue warnings about the safety of HRT.

As the population ages, there's been a trend to take hormone replacement whenever our bodies' natural supplies start to taper off. Findings suggesting effectiveness of hormone use for very limited applications—melatonin for jet lag, for instance, or testosterone replacement to restore muscle mass and libido in men with significant

What to Expect When . . .

Among the body's most powerful chemical agents, hormones orchestrate our stages of growth and physical change throughout our lifespan. Here are some of the key periods of hormone production and decline.

- **Teens:** Peak time for secretion of human growth hormone, which eventually dwindles from 1,000 to 1,500 micrograms to 50 micrograms produced each day.
- **Thirties:** Levels of DHEA (a hormone intermediate) peak. Most men begin a gradual, progressive decline in testosterone levels of about 1 percent a year.
- **Forties:** Most women become perimenopausal, a period of fluctuating hormone levels that can last several years. Forty-seven is the average age to start this phase.
- **Fifties:** Most women reach menopause (marked by the passage of a full year since the last period). Fifty-one is the average age and 45 to 55 the usual range.
- **Sixties and seventies:** Twenty percent of men measure below normal youthful testosterone levels. DHEA levels are significantly lower than before middle age.
- **Eighties:** Half of men measure below normal youthful testosterone levels.

deficiency—can fuel media headlines, which in turn fool consumers into believing advertisements that promote hormones as miracle treatments. However, we currently don't have the knowledge to use hormone supplements to restore or preserve youth, and taking them could cause you to age more, not less.

NEW HORMONE RULE #1
WOMEN, DON'T TAKE HORMONE REPLACEMENT UNLESS SEVERE MENOPAUSAL SYMPTOMS WARRANT IT

Imagine a pill that could protect you from heart attack, stroke, colon cancer, broken bones, and Alzheimer's disease; improve your memory, give you more energy; lower your cholesterol; help you sleep; and improve your sex life. How could you say no?

For about half of our 50-plus population, we believed that such a pill existed. It was called Premarin, estradiol, estrone, or other forms of estrogen. For the past couple of decades, estrogen looked like a godsend for postmenopausal women. Now, several important research findings have forced us to seriously question its use.

Over the past century, women's life expectancy has increased from 48 to 80 years, but the average onset of menopause remains unchanged at age 51. This means that a woman can expect to live an average of three decades after menopause. Little wonder that a pill that could relieve its symptoms would become one of the most widely prescribed medications in the country. In fact, before the announcement of the findings of the WHI, 38 percent of postmenopausal women were taking estrogen replacement therapy.

After adolescence and pregnancy, menopause is the next big hormonal event in a woman's life. Many women feel deeply derailed by mood swings, insomnia, hot flashes, night sweats, memory loss, diminished sex drive, and vaginal dryness. These symptoms can persist for many years—a long time to feel off your peak. When the 1960s brought the discovery that replacing lost estrogen could make most of these symptoms go away, doctors prescribed large doses and women happily popped the pills, thinking they could stay the hands of time.

Ten years later, in the 1970s, those same women were horrified when scientists discovered a link between estrogen replacement and increased risk of uterine cancer. Now estrogen was a carcinogen. Most doctors immediately quit writing prescriptions.

Still, the benefits of estrogen replacement seemed so desirable that scientists looked for a way around the problem, and by the 1980s they thought they had found it: Adding supplemental progestins (the synthetic form of progesterone) to estrogen eliminated the extra uterine cancer risk. I was the deputy director of the National Institute on Aging at the time, and we were very pleased with this news, since new data was pouring in that appeared to show even more advantages to estrogen replacement. It became clear that estrogen could help prevent osteoporosis, making it the first medication we had to reduce the incidence of hip fractures, a common cause of death and disability in older age. Furthermore, observational studies revealed that women who took HRT had lower risks of heart attack and stroke, risk of which skyrockets with menopause. Estrogen was back on the block.

By the 1990s doctors were trying out lower doses and new forms of HRT, personalizing each woman's prescription to maximize the benefits and minimize the side effects, such as headaches and breast tenderness, that came with the old higher doses. Meanwhile, findings continued to come out in HRT's favor. Observational studies showed that it might help prevent colon cancer, memory loss, and Alzheimer's disease. With such a simple and effective antidote to most of the serious age-related conditions seemingly at hand, sales of estrogen combination products soared.

If Maria had faced her decision about hormone replacement back in the 1990s, the answer would probably have been an easy yes. But today, results from better-controlled clinical trials are calling into question the findings of the observational studies. Study participants who take HRT tend to exercise more, smoke less, watch their weight, and eat better. These healthy lifestyle habits may well be what protects women on HRT from heart attacks, strokes, and Alzheimer's disease—not the hormones themselves. Only the data on estrogen's effect on menopausal symptoms such as hot flashes and protection against bone loss and colon cancer still look solid and unquestionable. Meanwhile, evidence for the risks of estrogen and progestin replacement continues to mount. In addition to the WHI's findings of increases in heart disease, stroke, pulmonary embolism, and breast cancer in the women who took HRT, other studies indicate an increased risk of ovarian cancer related to HRT. However, only one relatively high-dose combination of 0.625 milligrams conjugated equine estrogen (CEE), and 2.5 milligrams medroxyprogesterone acetate (MPA) was used in the WHI study and the Heart and Estrogen Replacement Study (HERS). It is possible that other estrogen and progestin combinations at lower dosage might not have these increased risks.

The Case for HRT

There are hopeful signs for hormone replacement on the horizon. Observational studies suggest that taking estrogen *might* help preserve cognition, prevent colon cancer, and protect against cataracts. We don't yet know whether these associations will unravel in controlled trials, so read enthusiastic media reports "with a grain of salt."

Memory loss: Estrogen may help improve the short-term memory loss that many menopausal women experience. Findings also suggest that HRT can improve verbal memory, reasoning, and motor speed for women suffering from symptoms of menopause. However, estrogen doesn't help brainpower where menopausal symptoms aren't present, suggesting that it may be relief from these distracting symptoms, and not the estrogen itself, that improves mental function.

Other data indicate that taking estrogen may help protect against Alzheimer's disease, one of the most dreaded specters of age. The first observational study linking previous estrogen use to protection against this devastating disease was done at our Andrus Gerontology Center here at the University of Southern California. Unfortunately, giving estrogen to patients who already have Alzheimer's doesn't slow the disease's progression.

Colon cancer: Another potential benefit of HRT is prevention of colon cancer. One in five women is affected by colon or rectal cancer during her lifetime, and preliminary data that HRT may reduce the risk for colon cancer offers hope for improving healthspan. A recent study by the Massachusetts Cancer Registry matched 515 female colorectal cancer patients with 515 controls (nonpatients) and found that recent HRT users were 40 percent less likely to develop colon cancer. The WHI also found decreased colon cancers in women taking HRT. A meta-analysis of 25 studies since 1966 found that women who used HRT reduced their risk of colon cancer by 12 to 33 percent. HRT use does not appear to protect against rectal cancer.

Cataracts: HRT could help keep you seeing well, too. Cataract surgery is the most frequent surgical procedure performed under Medicare—1.35 million operations per year—and postmenopausal women are the most likely candidates. Again, observational evidence suggests that HRT may help prevent cataracts, which cloud the eye's lens and can cause blindness unless surgically corrected.

The Framingham Eye Study, part of the larger Framington Heart Study, followed 529 women ranging in age from 66 to 93 and found that those who took HRT for 10 years or more reduced their risks of cataracts by 60 percent. However, as in other observational studies, the lifestyle of the subjects may have been a factor. The women taking HRT may also have eaten a healthy diet, including lots of fruits and vegetables, which can also prevent cataract formation.

The Case against HRT

We now know from the HERS and WHI studies that the reasons not to take HRT include increased risk of heart disease, stroke, breast cancer, gallbladder disease, and pulmonary embolism.

Heart disease: Before menopause, women enjoy greater natural protection from heart disease than men do, perhaps due to estrogen. After menopause, this advantage disappears, leaving women with roughly the same risk as men. Since estrogen replacement can lower LDL and raise HDL cholesterol, prime factors in heart disease, researchers postulated that HRT might help keep the heart healthy after menopause.

Most observational studies over the past few decades suggested this was true, as women taking HRT had less heart disease and fewer heart attacks than those who didn't. Then in 1998 came the results of HERS, the first randomized, double-blinded, placebo-controlled clinical trial of the effects of estrogen HRT on women with preexisting heart disease. The findings rocked the foundations of hormonal knowledge. These women had an *increased* risk of cardiovascular "events"—heart attack, stroke, or chest pains—in the first year on HRT, particularly the first 4 months. Those who stuck with HRT did see decreased risk of a heart attack by the fourth and fifth years of the trial, but unfortunately this is the time at which we start to observe increased risk of breast cancer.

With the findings of the WHI study confirming that HRT can increase the risk of heart attack, estrogens and progestins are no longer recommended for protection from cardiovascular disease.

Cancer and other risks: In addition to heart attack, hormone replacement therapy increases the risk of breast and ovarian cancer, as well as pulmonary embolism, stroke, thrombophlebitis (inflammation of veins that can lead to blood clots), gall bladder disease, and dry eyes. It can also have undesirable side effects such as breast tenderness and vaginal bleeding.

Breast tissue is densely populated with estrogen receptors, and a very significant downside of estrogen and progestin replacement is increased risk of breast cancer. A recent study of 40,000 menopausal women found that those on HRT had a 20 to 40 percent higher risk of breast cancer than those who didn't take estrogen, while a 2002 analysis of the data from a number of studies by the Collaborative Group on Hormonal Factors in Breast Cancer found that breast cancer incidence was 60 to 85 percent higher among recent long-term users of HRT. One of the main reasons the WHI was stopped in 2002 was the significantly increased risk of breast cancer in women taking estrogen-progestin supplements.

Time appears to be an important factor in the relationship between HRT and breast cancer. The shorter time you take hormone replacement, the less your risk. The good news is that stopping HRT within 5 years may return your risk to baseline—what it was before you started. The bad news is that longer use may leave you at higher risk even after you quit.

Extended use of HRT is also associated with ovarian cancer. The American Cancer Society's Cancer Prevention Study II followed 211,581 postmenopausal women for 14 years and found that those who used HRT for 10 years or more were 2.2 times more likely to get ovarian cancer. Ceasing HRT reduces risk but only by about half. Women who took HRT for 10-plus years and then quit had a 59 percent higher ovarian cancer risk. In a study of 44,000 postmenopausal women who took HRT over an extended period of time, long-term use was associated with an increasing risk of ovarian cancer. In fact with each additional year of HRT, the risk increased by 7 percent.

NEW HORMONE RULE #2:
WOMEN, CONSIDER ESTROGEN ALTERNATIVES, BUT WISELY

The risks of hormone replacement therapy are leading scientists to search for alternatives. At the forefront of these investigations are a new class of medications known as selective estrogen receptor modulators (SERMs) and estrogen-like compounds found in plants, called phytoestrogens.

SERMs

The recent discovery of SERMs may offer many women a significant edge on successful aging. SERMs are drugs that bind to cell receptors for estrogen to act like proestrogens in bones and blood, but block estrogen receptors in breast tissue to have an anti-estrogen effect. This means that SERMs can protect bone density without increasing cancer risk. In fact the first SERM to take the spotlight, tamoxifen, is now used as a highly effective treatment for breast cancer.

We're now working on the second generation of SERMs, and the leading drug, raloxifene (trade name Evista), may rewrite old rules to end up in the New Rules canon. Not only does raloxifene increase bone mineral density and reduce the risk of breast cancer, but for certain women it could also cut the risk of cardiovascular events. In the Multiple Outcomes of Raloxifene Evaluation Trial, a 5-year study of 7,705 post-menopausal women with osteoporosis, participants at increased risk for heart disease (defined as having high blood pressure, diabetes, elevated blood lipids, previous heart disease, or smoking cigarettes) were 40 percent less likely to suffer a cardiovascular event when taking raloxifene.

The tradeoffs of taking raloxifene include increased risk of thromboembolism (blood clots), which is also a downside of estrogen, and this drug doesn't control hot flashes. On balance, raloxifene represents a very viable alternative for women in later life who need protection against bone loss and heart disease.

Phytoestrogens

In the search for estrogen alternatives, many women look to Mother Earth. Estrogen-like compounds occur naturally in a number of plants, including isoflavones in soybeans, coumestans in clover and alfalfa sprouts, and lignans in flaxseed. These phytoestrogens (*phyto-* means "plant") are held up as a beacon of hope by those who prefer not to take pharmaceutical estrogen or SERMs. Do these natural chemicals have the same protective benefits of estrogen without the risks, or are phytoestrogens a product of wishful thinking?

At the moment, we don't know. The phytoestrogens in soy, called isoflavones, are similar in structure and function to estrogen, but like SERMs, they pick and choose which estrogen receptors to connect with or block, and they seem to make smart choices. Isoflavones act as antiestrogens in breast and uterine tissue but proestrogens in blood and bones. Theoretically, isoflavones could provide health benefits to women during and after menopause without increasing cancer risk.

The outlook for phytoestrogens was exciting at first. In a pattern that's familiar by now if you've read the preceding chapters of this book, observational studies of Asian populations initially suggested that a soy-rich diet may provide the best of estrogen and anti-estrogen effects: protection against cardiovascular disease; breast, prostate, and colon cancer; bone loss; and the symptoms of menopause. Unfortunately, intervention studies have yet to prove these postulates true.

The effects of phytoestrogens are weak compared to estrogen or SERM therapy, and the limited data that we have suggests that, at best, eating a lot of soy may:

- Moderately attenuate bone loss
- Lower total and LDL cholesterol, though the effect on heart disease risk is not known
- Slightly relieve the symptoms of menopause, but far less effectively than estrogen

Until we have long-term research on the effects of phytoestrogen exposure, it's not time to take isoflavone supplements. Isoflavones isolates may not contain the natural compounds found in soy foods and could even turn out to be harmful. For now, feel free to enjoy moderate amounts of whole soy foods in your healthy diet. But don't overdo it, hoping to replace lost estrogen. There's not enough evidence in their favor and we know little about the risks of high consumption.

Making Your Decision

There remains only one good reason to consider HRT: relief from severe symptoms of menopause. Many women who take estrogen during this volatile time feel that they regain life as they knew it—a precious gift, plain and simple though it may seem. So if you've tried everything and still are plagued by extreme symptoms, you might consider HRT. But weigh your risks carefully.

Protection against osteoporosis, on the other hand, no longer presents a good case for HRT. While estrogen can protect against bone loss, the protection lasts only as long as you take it, and the risks of long-term use are too high. Now we have other highly effective treatments for osteoporosis, so HRT needn't even be an option.

To help guide your decision about how to handle the onset of menopause, consult the "Comparison of Estrogen, Raloxifene, and Phytoestrogens" table on the next page. Here you'll find a list of treatment alternatives for the symptoms and risks of menopause that can help you select a strategy that best addresses your personal health issues.

Once you've surveyed your options, schedule an appointment to discuss them with your doctor. (It may be your internist, gynecologist, or cardiologist.) If your doctor doesn't have the time to discuss this important issue with you, find another physician who will! You deserve a supportive guide to help you make your decision.

Take this book to your appointment with the page for "Comparison of Estrogen, Raloxifene, and Phytoestrogens" marked, your own list of personal questions and concerns, and paper and pen for taking notes. Don't leave the office until you've discussed every issue and noted your doctor's response and any other thoughts that arise.

If you choose to try short-term HRT, your decision-making process may have just begun. Hormone replacement has side effects that make some women uncomfortable. If you aren't happy with how HRT makes you feel, work with your doctor to explore different prescriptions and

Don't Put Your Love Life on Pause

Changes to the vaginal lining during menopause can cause dryness and painful sex. This can be effectively treated with topical estrogen creams that carry none of the risks of estrogen pills.

Comparison of Estrogen, Raloxifene, and Phytoestrogens

Here are all your options for treating menopause at a glance.

Benefit/Risk	Estrogen	Raloxifene (Evista)	Phytoestrogens	Other Alternatives
Bone mineral density	Very good increase	Good increase	Little to no effect	Bisphosphonates (Fosamax), weight-bearing exercise, strength training
Cardiovascular disease risk	Slightly increased	May reduce	May reduce	Diet, exercise, weight management
Total and LDL cholesterol levels	Lowered	Lowered	Lowered somewhat	Diet, exercise, weight management
Thromboembolism risk	Increased	Increased	None	
Breast cancer risk	Increased	Decreased	Not clear	
Ovarian cancer risk	Increased	Not clear	Not clear	
Uterine cancer risk	Increased if given without progesterone	None	Not clear	Not clear
Hot flashes and other symptoms of menopause	Relieves	Can make worse	Little to no effect	Clonidine, Paxil, black cohosh, vitamin E, vaginal estrogen creams

doses. One option is to administer the hormones by patch, which bypasses the liver and prevents certain side effects. It's also important to choose the time horizon for hormone replacement. My New Rule is to take *the lowest dose possible for the shortest time possible to minimize your exposure to risk.*

Whatever your age, I encourage you to visit www.longevityquotient.com to stay up to date on menopause management and to regularly reevaluate your situation in light of current information and your own health indicators.

MEN, DON'T TAKE TESTOSTERONE UNLESS YOUR DOCTOR RECOMMENDS IT

Testosterone, the male counterpart to estrogen, fuels sex drive and helps to maintain muscle mass and bone strength. Unlike estrogen, however, testosterone doesn't decline abruptly with age. In their thirties, many men begin to experience a gradual, progressive decline in testosterone levels at an average rate of about 1 percent per year. By age 60, about 20 percent of men are below normal testosterone levels for healthy young men, and the number has grown to 50 percent of us by age 80. In some men, testosterone levels don't diminish at all. This represents a much less dramatic and more variable change than faced by the female population. Though we don't know precisely what factors cause testosterone loss, possible ones include genes, excess weight, poor diet, alcohol or tobacco use, stress, and medical conditions. AgeLess living can help you avoid all of these factors except for genetics.

Male Menopause, Fact or Fiction?

Is male menopause a medical fact? When she was researching her book *Male Passages*, author Gail Sheehy asked me that. Actually, the word "passage" is a much better word to describe men's midlife hormonal shifts. There's no direct male counterpart for the precipitous estrogen drop-off that women experience in menopause. But midlife can bring noticeable physiological and psychological effects related to diminishing levels of testosterone. Many men feel that they've entered a new, less youthful stage of life.

Age-related decline in testosterone levels can cause symptoms that include loss of muscle strength along with increased body fat, low energy and stamina, reduced sexual drive and/or function, and depressed mood. When testosterone levels dip below the normal range for young men and the decline is accompanied by one or more of these symptoms, doctors call the condition testosterone deficiency. But because these changes are, medically speaking, much more limited in degree and intensity than the ones women experience during menopause, most doctors don't consider the male menopause metaphor apt. Whether or not to treat testosterone deficiency in older men remains a question of medical debate.

Testosterone Replacement Does Not Pass the New Rules Test—Yet

In young men who are genetically deficient in the hormone, testosterone replacement is very effective in boosting libido, increasing muscle mass, and lowering cholesterol. For men middle-aged and above whose testosterone levels have declined below the youthful range of normal, it can be tempting to get a quick injection in hopes of recovering your firm biceps and sexual fire—but you probably shouldn't. Taking supplementary testosterone increases your risk of a heart attack, the biggest threat to your healthspan. Testosterone replacement can also enlarge the prostate and may increase your prostate cancer risk. In fact, one of the ways doctors treat advanced prostate cancer is with (brace yourself) castration to remove testosterone from your bloodstream or with chemicals that block the hormone's effects (indelicately known as chemical castration). Do you really want to take a hormone that feeds prostate cancer cells?

The few studies of testosterone replacement in older men have found some increases in libido, mood, muscle mass, and bone mineral density—but these benefits are outweighed by the risks. This unrealized potential is what keeps scientists looking for a way to safely replace testosterone. There are a number of studies under way, supported by the National Institute on Aging, that should provide more information and map the route for the future.

Testosterone replacement is only available through prescription, but the pill form of testosterone is never a good idea, since the hormone can damage your liver as it passes through during digestion. Instead, knowledgeable doctors prescribe skin patches or injections that bypass the digestive process.

Also watch for SARMs, or selective androgen receptor modulators, which are currently under development. Similar to SERMs, these drugs work on cell receptors for testosterone to, it is hoped, provide the benefits of the hormone (increased libido, bone density, and muscle strength and improved mood) without the risks of heart disease and prostate cancer.

Stop by www.longevityquotient.com to stay abreast of testosterone news. In the meantime, eat right, pump iron, and get plenty of sleep to make the most of the testosterone you've got.

Test Your TQ—Testosterone Quotient

Could you be testosterone deficient? Answer "yes" or "no" to the following questions to gauge where you stand.

1. Do you have diminished sexual drive? _____
2. Do you have decreased energy? _____
3. Do you have decreased strength? _____
4. Have you lost weight? _____
5. Have you noticed decreased enjoyment of life? _____
6. Are you frequently sad or grumpy? _____
7. Are your erections less strong? _____
8. Has your ability to play sports decreased? _____
9. Do you fall asleep after dinner? _____
10. Has your work performance deteriorated? _____

If you answered "yes" to number 1 or 7 or to three or more questions total, I recommend talking with your doctor about testing your testosterone levels.

Adapted from: John Morley, "Testosterone Replacement and the Physiologic Aspects of Aging in Men." In *Mayo Clinic Proceedings*, Volume 75 Supplement, January 2000, S83–S87

NEW HORMONE RULE #4:

JUST SAY "NO" TO HUMAN GROWTH HORMONE, DHEA, ANDROSTENEDIONE, AND MELATONIN

These days, you can't open your mail, read the paper, or surf the Web without finding a spate of claims for hormones purported to make you age less. As lovely as the prospect sounds, don't believe the hype. We don't have the hormone of eternal youth—at least not yet. Here is the truth about some of the fake contenders:

HGH

Back in 1990, the news media broadcast far and wide the findings from a small study of 21 elderly men in Wisconsin. These participants increased muscle and bone strength, lost fat, and regained the skin of 50-year-olds with a mere 6 months of HGH treatment. The HGH craze was on.

As its name suggests, HGH stimulates normal growth of bones, muscles, and tissues in children. At the age of 13 and in the midst of a huge growth spurt, my son is awash in HGH; his levels are probably 10 or 20 times higher than mine. While he's excited to measure his height each month and watch himself shoot to the sky, he also complains of pains in his hips, legs, and knees. These literal growing pains are a normal part of adolescence caused by rapid growth during this time. By contrast, children with a rare medical condition that makes them deficient in HGH will not develop to normal height without hormone treatment.

As you might expect, when you stop growing, your HGH levels taper off, from secretions of about 1,000 to 1,500 micrograms a day during pubescence to as little as 50 micrograms per day in your sixties. In other words, you end up with about 5 percent of the HGH you had as a teen. This decline is accompanied by loss of bone density and muscle mass and the development of abdominal fat. What can we do about it? Obviously, take HGH—it sounds like a no-brainer, doesn't it?

Certainly, that's what all those e-mail advertisers and antiaging clinics want you to think when you consider their invitations: Take HGH to stay fit, strong, and trim forever! Reduce body fat and build muscle without exercise. Enhance sexual performance, remove wrinkles and cellulite, restore hair color and growth, strengthen your immune system, turn back your biological clock by 20 years!

Sound too good to be true? It is. Unfortunately, the facts don't support the fantasy; not even close. Since that 1990 study, countless controlled clinical trials have failed to confirm the miraculous results of HGH replacement. This was not for lack of trying. Researchers have hunted for the supposed benefits of HGH in men and women alike and found little evidence that growth hormone supplements do anything to slow down the aging process or that a decline in growth hormone levels is a major contributor to age-related bone and muscle loss. Meanwhile, there are clear risks to taking HGH: diabetes and carpal tunnel syndrome.

Some legitimate cases do call for growth hormone therapy—children who aren't growing at a normal rate and adults with growth hormone deficiency related to pituitary disease. There have been some interesting findings suggesting that growth hormone supplements can reduce abdominal fat in older men, which could theoretically "trim" the risk of heart disease, high cholesterol and blood pressure, and insulin insensitivity. But no one has actually proven that such fat removal reduces disease risk, and women who take HGH don't seem to enjoy this belly-busting benefit.

In any case, replacing missing HGH is easier said than done. The medical community has yet to agree upon a good way to assess growth hormone deficiency or to match specific low hormone levels to appropriate treatment strengths. And you'll need to grow your bank account before you take up growth hormone treatment. The annual cost is around $10,000. Income from these treatments is a mainstay of many antiaging clinics.

For now, no one should take growth hormone supplements simply to combat the effects of age. The best ways we know to optimize your natural HGH secretions are to stay active, watch your weight if you're gaining abdominal fat, and get plenty of sleep.

DHEA

Another common acronym in the antiaging trade is DHEA, or dehydroepiandrosterone. (You see why the nickname caught on.) A steroid formed in the production of male and female sex hormones, DHEA seems to have gained its sexy reputation by association. However, there's no evidence to support claims that taking DHEA restores amour, melts away love handles, bolsters lagging energy, or lengthens lives.

Luckily, consumers have largely caught on. Where health food store windows once displayed large-lettered signs shouting WE HAVE DHEA, you can now buy remaindered stock at a deep discount. How did it become the rage in the first place?

DHEA is abundant in the body, second only to cholesterol in its concentrations, so it would seem to make sense that it's there to do something. Levels of DHEA peak sometime between ages 25 and 35, then begin a steady decline that leaves you at a significantly lower level by age 60. You definitely lose DHEA as you age.

Research on mice fueled the initial excitement about DHEA as an antidote for age. I collaborated on this early animal research with the famous French scientist Dr. Etienne Baulieu, also known for inventing RU-486 (the morning-after birth control pill) and being the lover of Sophia Loren. I remember well a warm summer day by the pool in the Foxhall Road district of Washington, D.C., with Dr. Baulieu and the lovely Ms. Loren when we discussed findings that treating mice with DHEA could prevent certain cancers, diabetes, and other age-related conditions. As a young researcher, I was certainly energized by the possibilities, though I may have been a little starstruck, too.

Subsequent studies suggested that old mice on DHEA had improved immune function. Supplement manufacturers caught wind of these tantalizing findings and started hawking DHEA pills to people.

Unfortunately, not all of the mouse claims have held up as well over the years as Sophia Loren has, and attempts to duplicate them in humans have roundly failed. A number of well-designed clinical studies have administered DHEA to older people with low levels of the hormone and found no discernible effect on body fat, strength, sense of well-being, sexual function, or anything else you might want to improve with age. Other studies have found no consistent relationship between DHEA levels and heart disease or overall mortality. The evidence that taking DHEA can prevent age-related complaints simply doesn't exist.

What we do have is the possibility of side effects ranging from undesirable to dangerous. Since the body can convert DHEA to both estrogen and testosterone, taking supplements can raise your risk of breast or prostate cancer. DHEA can also spur unwanted hair growth on body and face as well as cause acne, an attribute of adolescence most of us are all too happy to leave behind.

Perhaps the day will come when we find proof for benefits of DHEA supplements that outweigh the risks. Until then, pitch those DHEA pills and resist the urge to buy the discounted leftovers languishing on the shelves.

Androstenedione

In 1998, St. Louis Cardinal outfielder Mark McGwire electrified America by breaking the 37-year-old home run record of Yankee Roger Maris, who outdid the legendary Babe Ruth. Almost overnight McGwire's favorite supplement, androstenedione, sparked a major controversy. Doctors lamented the lack of evidence for andro's safety and effectiveness, but the public didn't seem to care. If a pill was giving McGwire superhuman ability, bring it on! Among the crowds lining up to buy androstenedione were plenty of men in rebellion against the way age and inactivity were robbing them of muscle mass.

Alas, androstenedione is probably not the answer. It is a precursor steroid, which means that the compound can be converted in the body to both testosterone and estrogen, and some believe andro can serve as a natural alternative to chemical steroids to build muscle size and strength. However, the few controlled studies that have been conducted show no such benefit. The list of potential risks, however, is long: heart attack, prostate cancer, decreased good (HDL) cholesterol, acne, and male pattern baldness. Women on andro may experience a new crop of body hair and a deeper voice.

The Olympic Committee and other sports organizations have since banned androstenedione. Though this might be taken as proof that it enhances sports performance, the ban is probably not protecting fair competition, although it may help guard athletes' health. I recommend that you say "no" to andro.

Melatonin

Another popular topic for the books touting miracle cures for age is melatonin, a hormone that helps regulate our day-night cycles. The enthusiasm began when some Italian investigators found that giving melatonin to old mice made them act like young mice again. However, many people excited about the news did not know that these mice had genetically low levels of melatonin to begin with. When older mice with normal melatonin levels were given melatonin supplements, they showed no age-related changes. So much for the so-called miracle.

Your pineal gland secretes melatonin in response to signals from your eyes about exposure to light and dark. Melatonin secretion peaks at night to signal the brain and body that it's time to go to sleep. This has led to some speculation that low melatonin levels might account for age-related sleep loss as well as other "unspecified" signs of aging. Might it then follow that melatonin supplements can restore healthy sleep and other youthful attributes? Probably not. Age-related sleep loss doesn't appear to be due to any drop in melatonin levels. Older people make plenty of the stuff. Furthermore, melatonin has proven to be a poor sleep medication, and people who take it show no other signs of aging less.

Still, you might not want to throw your melatonin stash away. This supplement can be helpful for resetting your body clock to compensate for jet lag, early weekday mornings after late-night weekends, night shift work, or for blind individuals who don't respond to cycles of light and dark with appropriate melatonin secretion.

Do I have a miracle cure for age? Sure. You can read all about it in the other chapters of this book. Eat right, watch your weight, exercise and pump iron, get a good night's sleep, and engage in life. Ignore the testimonials for over-the-counter hormones and supplements and run, don't walk, away from any claim using the word "miracle."

HAVE AN AGELESS DAY
Hormones

Still thinking about hormones? Think again. These AgeLess sleep, exercise, and diet activities give hormones a natural boost.

- **Get up** at the same time each morning to regularize secretion of melatonin.
- **Toss out** your HGH, DHEA, androstenedione, and isoflavone supplements. Don't beg your doctor for testosterone.
- **Work out.** An aerobic workout followed by a weight-lifting session can provide many of the benefits of estrogen, testosterone, and growth hormone without the risks.
- **Enjoy soy.** Sure, have some tofu in that stir-fry! Moderate amounts of soy are part of a longevity diet for men and women alike—but don't expect antiaging miracles.
- **Reassess.** If you're taking HRT, now is the time to assess the need and duration of its use and consider possible alternatives. Sit down and write your list of pros, cons, questions, and concerns. Make an appointment to discuss them with your doctor.
- **Sleep tight!** Get a good night's sleep to maximize secretion of HGH and boost your energy in the world's most natural way.

CHAPTER 8

SHOPPING FOR LONGEVITY

I ONCE ACTED AS SCIENTIFIC ADVISOR to an investigative reporter for a major television network for a story about self-proclaimed rejuvenation clinics that promised to reverse aging. His assignment was to check in as a patient to these facilities all over the world and report on their treatments.

One night the phone rang in my office. It was the reporter calling from a spa in Switzerland. The next morning, he was scheduled to have an injection of fetal sheep cells. Understandably, he was worried. What were the safety implications of this ovine booster shot?

I assured the correspondent that the shot was probably completely harmless—and totally ineffective. It would do nothing to delay his aging process. I couldn't resist poking fun at him—I told him that the worst that could happen would be that he'd develop an allergy to lamb chops. You'll be far better off, I said, enjoying some real AgeLess rejuvenation—getting a good night's sleep.

When the TV show aired, it covered scores of similarly outlandish claims, along with the real news: The reporter found little to no evidence that any of these treatments actually worked. Of course, such mythbusting stories are broadcast all the time, but business remains brisk in the longevity industry anyway. Why do we continue to hold out hope that one of these fixes might eventually "cure" aging? The fact is that our hope to find the fountain of youth never dies.

New Buzzwords, Old Quest

In ancient Egypt, the pharaohs devoted enormous resources building pyramids meant to ensure that they would live eternal lives beyond this earthly one. The Greek myths are full of humans seeking immortality, and a lucky few actually succeeded. But even the ancient Greeks under-stood that without good health, eternal life was a tragic folly. When the goddess Enyo went to Zeus, king of the gods, to request immortality for her mortal lover, Tithonos, she forgot to ask for perpetual youth, too. Enyo was gravely disappointed to find herself stuck with a continuously aging old man for a boyfriend.

In the 16th century, the Spanish adventurer Ponce de León heard stories of a famous spring that had the power to restore youth and vigor to those who drank its waters. Off he sailed for what is now southern Florida. If you went there today, you might think that his "fountain of youth" had the opposite effect. A hundred years ago, hucksters roamed the country in covered wagons selling "snake oil," patent medicines (made mostly of alcohol), and other wares promising health and youth.

Today, the sales pitches are more sophisticated. The rich and famous pay thousands of dollars to travel to exclusive getaways for treatments with names like body cleansing, chelation therapy, and hyperbaric oxygen therapy—but the promises remain mostly false. We of more modest means may go to our local health food stores to stock up on melatonin, a hormone touted as an antiaging miracle in several best-selling books, or belly up to the local oxygen bar hoping that a hit of pure O_2 can increase alertness, enhance physical performance, and im-prove the body's ability to burn fat better than the air in the living room. Never mind that at rest our blood is usually over 97 percent saturated with oxygen and it's hard to improve on this level.

The Tower of Babel: How to Make Sense of Claims for Eternal Youth and Beauty

I've seen products that promise longevity sometimes tempting otherwise reasonable people to shop until they drop. We'd all like to stop the rav-ages of aging, and in the information age, we're bombarded with claims for products and services that promise to help. You can't read a maga-zine or watch TV, surf the Net, talk with colleagues and friends, go to the gym, hit the health food store, or even walk the supermarket aisles without facing a barrage of ads and advice.

Even the most health-conscious shopper can have a hard time making sense of the noise coming from this modern-day Tower of Babel. What and whom should you believe? As a consumer, you're at a great disadvantage when it comes to evaluating health information. It's not like buying a car, where you can go to the library and pick up a copy of *Consumer Reports* or visit any number of reputable Web sites to do research. Nor are there many state or federal laws that protect you from inaccurate and misleading health claims.

Adding to the burden may be your own fears about aging. As those wrinkles multiply, who wouldn't want to believe an infomercial "expert" who cites a "scientific breakthrough" or buy the antiaging lotion that makes a 20-year-old model's skin look flawless? Some companies aren't shy about trying to get you to buy their products by making them look and sound like another one. After Viagra became an overnight sensation, Internet companies marketed sexual potency products with the copycat names Vaegra and Viagro. Though the maker of Viagra stopped the copycats by filing trademark infringement suits, plenty of companies willing to prey on consumer confusion are still busily plying their trade.

How to Spot False Claims

Here are a few simple ways to detect sham experts and false claims. Watch for these red flags, then run away as fast as you can:

- **"Miracles," "cures," and "breakthroughs."** You didn't see Louis Pasteur write a book called *The Smallpox Miracle* or Jonas Salk promoting a "Cure Polio at Home!" kit. Most health books and products using the words miracle, cure, or breakthrough are created by swindlers, not scientists.
- **Detoxification and cleansing.** You do not need to detoxify or cleanse your body. As Jane Brody, longtime health writer for the *New York Times*, points out, "You have a liver for that." Most so-called cleansing treatments are enemas, which are uncomfortable and usually expensive procedures involving liquid going the wrong way in a very private part of your body. There's no evidence that such cleansing is beneficial to your health or that it's even safe.
- **Single solutions—the "magic bullet."** Aging is a very complex biological process, and it's unlikely that a single cause will ever be found. Certainly, no single solution exists that we know of today. Our current understanding is that aging is the result of many different genes interacting with various environmental

factors. Don't believe claims that one pill or one technique will turn back the clock.

Interpreting Scientific Studies

Even information from legitimate scientific experts can sometimes get quite confusing. For instance, many nutrition experts recommend that you cut back on fat, despite the abundant evidence that omega-3 and monounsaturated fats are good for you. Researchers can point to statistics showing that some smokers never develop lung cancer. Does this mean that cigarettes are safe?

Unless you've been trained to interpret studies, you can easily draw the wrong conclusions from studies published in prestigious scientific publications. One study published in *JAMA*, a leading medical journal, found that men with the most fat in their diet had a lower risk of strokes from blood clots. Taking the results of this article on face value, you might return to those steaks and Häagen-Dazs with relish. But if you review more of the scientific literature, you'll see that this finding completely opposes the vast body of evidence linking increased saturated fat intake with higher risks of heart and blood vessel disease. If you look at the article closely, you might find that the way the study was conducted does not justify drawing conclusions about fat intake and stroke. And because it's part of our jobs as scientists to place our work in context, then frame the *next* set of questions, it's likely that the studies's authors advised such caution; unfortunately the press doesn't always bother to read the fine print. Such disclaimers rarely make it to the headlines.

Judging Natural Products

Mother Nature did a great job of providing most of the things we need for health and longevity. The New Rules outlined in this book rely mostly on natural practices to expand your healthspan. However, in the hyped-up world of health products, natural is not always better.

"Natural" is a buzzword that manufacturers apply to everything from foods to pills to makeup, often in a bid to boost the price tag. There are two problems with the premise that natural is always better. The first is that sometimes a synthetic alternative does the job as well or better. For instance, while I firmly advocate a natural approach to nutrition based on food, we can actually synthesize a better, more absorbable form of the critical nutrient folate in the lab than any you'll find in nature.

The second concern is more serious. Nature is full of toxins: arsenic, lead, foxglove, cyanide—all natural, all deadly. Ephedra is a popular natural herbal diet aid associated with health risks and death. Calcium purified from natural sources usually contains lead. To meet federal and state lead-safety standards, manufacturers have to treat it chemically. Don't turn off your common sense just because you see "natural" on the label. Rattlesnake venom is natural, too.

Reining In Our Enthusiasm

As a nation, we're exuberant people. We like to work hard, play hard, and do many things to extremes. We tend to think that if a little bit of something is good, a lot will be sublime. Most of the time this isn't true.

Supplements of *any* kind, even those sold over the counter, should be treated like drugs. Your body can only absorb so much of a substance at a time. Taking more than that is a waste, leading mainly to more expensive urine. Sometimes it can be quite dangerous. Many nutrients, from vitamin D to calcium, are necessary to life but become toxic at very high doses. Don't megadose on supplements, period. (See chapter 2 for more information on nutritional supplements.)

Shopping for Longevity

I hope that if you've learned anything from this book it's that most of you are better served by closing your wallets and following the holistic AgeLess program. In fact, one of the major findings about aging is that the best way to promote healthy lifespan is with an integrated lifestyle plan. In the sections that follow, I'll help you translate what you've learned in previous chapters into a few "best of the best" decisions.

A Consumer's Guide to AgeLess Products

You can buy all sorts of supplements that promise to slow, reverse, or cure aging. The question is, should you? And if so, which ones? I've created the AgeLess Shopping List on page 228 to guide you through the confusing maze and make shopping for longevity simple and—this is important—safe.

The AgeLess Shopping List covers the most popular longevity supplements and divides them into three categories:

⑥ **What Works:** These are products that have proven to be effective and relatively safe in repeated, well-conducted, scientific studies. They've earned the Dean's seal of approval.

⑥ **The Jury Is Out:** In this category, you'll find products for which the evidence is mixed. Some studies have suggested that they work while others cast doubt. I don't generally recommend these supplements at this time, though some individuals may have reason to take them.

⑥ **Don't Bother:** Promoted with much more hype than fact, these are the supplements you're likely to see in overstated advertisements. There are few if any good studies to support the use or safety of these products, and I don't recommend them.

The AgeLess Shopping List
What Works

You can put these items on your shopping list for longevity with confidence and the Dean's endorsement.

Buy?	Item	Claim	Truth
✓	Baby aspirin	Reduces risk of heart disease and colon cancer	Many studies confirm aspirin's ability to prevent heart attacks and colon cancer. In some individuals, aspirin can cause stomach and intestinal bleeding and distress. **The Dean's Recommendation: If you're at risk for heart disease, ask your doctor about taking one baby aspirin a day.**
✓	Calcium	Strengthens bones Prevents colon cancer Lowers blood pressure Prevents heart disease	Believe the claims. Many clinical studies support the need for adequate intake of calcium. **The Dean's Recommendation: 1,000 to 1,500 milligrams of calcium a day from diet and supplements (see chapter 2).**
✓	Folic acid	Prevents heart disease Reduces the risk of colon cancer	The claims are true. Increasing evidence supports the need for adequate intake of folic acid. **The Dean's Recommendation: 800 micrograms of folic acid a day from diet and supplements (see chapter 2).**

Buy?	Item	Claim	Truth
✓	Omega-3 fatty acids from fish	Reduce risk of death by stabilizing heart's electrical system	We know that eating omega-3 fatty acids in fish reduces deaths from heart disease. More studies are needed to confirm the benefits of omega-3 fatty acid pills. **The Dean's Recommendation: Have two servings of fatty fish per week (see chapter 2).**
✓	Vitamin D	Helps body to absorb calcium May prevent certain cancers	D is the number one vitamin deficiency in America, particularly in northern latitudes during winter. **The Dean's Recommendation: 1,000 IU of vitamin D a day from sunshine, food, and supplements (many calcium supplements also contain vitamin D; see chapter 2). Don't overdo supplements, as too much vitamin D can be toxic.**

The Jury Is Out

There's not enough evidence to earn a Dean's recommendation for taking these supplements. Individual variables may affect your own decision.

Buy?	Item	Claim	Truth
?	Multivitamins	Provide daily requirements for vitamins, minerals, and other micronutrients	**Good:** Multivitamins provide some folic acid, calcium, and vitamin D. **Bad:** They provide a false sense of security and don't provide enough of vital nutrients. **Ugly:** Many multivitamins contain unneeded and potentially dangerously high levels of vitamin A and iron. **The Dean's Recommendation: Toss out your multivitamin, eat right, and take the right doses of a few select supplements (see chapter 2).**
?	Vitamin C	Prevents heart disease, cancer, cataracts, and the common cold Antioxidant that slows the aging process	There's good scientific support for the benefits of vitamin C from foods, including protection against heart disease, stroke, some cancers, and cataracts. There's less evidence that vitamin C supplements have these same effects. **The Dean's Recommendation: Get 250 daily milligrams of vitamin C from your diet (see chapter 2).**

Buy?	Item	Claim	Truth
?	Vitamin E	Reduces risk of heart disease, stroke, cancer, and Alzheimer's disease Antioxidant that slows the aging process	When ingested in foods, vitamin E may reduce the risk of heart disease and have other health benefits, too. However, well-controlled studies of vitamin E supplements don't show any consistent effect on heart disease. It's hard to get much vitamin E in your diet, so the supplement decision is hard to call. **The Dean's Recommendation: Get as much vitamin E from your diet as you can. If you take a vitamin E supplement, it should not be more than 400 mg.**

Don't Bother

The following products probably won't help and in some cases may harm your healthspan. Leave your money in your pocket; I don't recommend them.

Buy?	Item	Claim	Truth
✗	Alpha lipoic acid	Antioxidant promoted for health and longevity	There's no evidence that alpha lipoic acid improves health or longevity in humans **The Dean's Recommendation: Don't take alpha lipoic acid.**
✗	Beta-carotene	Prevents heart disease, strokes, and cancer	Eating foods that contain beta-carotene can protect you from heart disease, strokes, and certain cancers. However, studies of beta-carotene supplements show that they do nothing to protect your healthspan and may even increase your risk of cancer. **The Dean's Recommendation: Eat plenty of fruits and vegetables containing beta-carotene but do not take beta-carotene supplements (see chapter 2).**
✗	Chelation therapy (A series of intravenous infusions containing disodium EDTA)	Treats accumulation of toxic metals in your body to prevent and treat heart disease and slow down aging	There is no scientific justification for this therapy. Among the metals removed by EDTA is calcium, which is important for strong bones and for preventing heart disease and colon cancer. **The Dean's Recommendation: Do not have chelation therapy.**

Buy?	Item	Claim	Truth
✗	Choline	Increases brainpower	There's no evidence that choline improves brain function. **The Dean's Recommendation: Don't take choline supplements.**
✗	Coenzyme Q_{10}	Antioxidant that stops aging and improves heart function	While coenzyme Q_{10} does have antioxidant properties, it offers no great advantage over fruits and vegetables or vitamins C and E. **The Dean's Recommendation: Eat plenty of fruits and vegetables and don't take coenzyme Q.**
✗	Deprenyl	Slows brain aging Treats Parkinson's disease	Deprenyl has had modest success in treating Parkinson's disease but does not affect aging. **The Dean's Recommendation: Do not take deprenyl unless a physician prescribes it for Parkinson's disease.**
✗	DHEA	Increases immune function Protects against heart disease Prevents cancer Increases lean body mass Improves well-being	DHEA has not been shown to live up to any of its promoters' claims and may increase risk of breast and prostate cancer. **The Dean's Recommendation: Don't take DHEA (see chapter 7).**
✗	Estrogen replacement	Helps menopausal symptoms Prevents osteoporosis and fractures Reduces risk of heart disease and strokes Prevents Alzheimer's disease	While estrogen does help relieve menopausal symptoms and reduces the risk of osteoporosis, recent studies indicate that the risks outweigh the benefits. Estrogen and progestin increase the risk of breast cancer, strokes, pulmonary embolism, gallstones, and ovarian cancer. **The Dean's Recommendation: Look for alternatives and try to avoid taking hormone replacement. If you must take estrogen, limit its use to as short a period as possible.**

Buy?	Item	Claim	Truth
✗	Gerovital, GH3	Long promoted as an anti-aging drug, now up-dated with additional ingredients and now called GH3	Gerovital is a form of procaine, a local anesthetic. It has no other effects except as a weak antidepressant. **The Dean's Recommendation: Don't take Gerovital or GH3.**
✗	Ginseng	Increases sexuality and brainpower	Though it's long been treasured by Asian cultures, there's no evidence that ginseng does anything for health or longevity. **The Dean's Recommendation: Don't take ginseng.**
✗	Human growth hormone (HGH)	Increases muscle strength Reduces body fat Builds bone density Improves vigor	While some studies show that HGH may promote loss of abdominal fat, other results are less consistent. This very expensive treatment ($10,000 or more) requires multiple injections and increases the risk of diabetes and carpal tunnel syndrome. **The Dean's Recommendation: Don't take HGH until more good studies support its use.**
✗	L-carnitine	Improves heart health and circulation Increases energy Improves brain function	L-carnitine has been found to help thyroid disease, Peyronie's disease, peripheral vascular disease, childhood liver disease, and dialysis patients. This will be an interesting compound to watch for future studies of aging and age-related diseases. **The Dean's Recommendation: For now, don't take L-carnitine unless you have one of the conditions described above and then, under medical supervision.**
✗	Lycopene, lutein, and zeaxanthin	Antioxidants that reduce risk of heart disease, prostate cancer, cataracts, and macular degeneration	These carotenoids (a class of antioxidants), plentiful in fruits and vegetables, are great for health and longevity when eaten in food, but there's no evidence that they have any effect as supplement pills. **The Dean's Recommendation: Get your lycopene, lutein, and zeaxanthin from vegetables and fruits, not pills.**

Buy?	Item	Claim	Truth
✗	Melatonin	Helps to reset the pineal gland and endocrine system to produce a "youthful" hormonal balance and regulatory cycle Aids sleep	Melatonin has no effect on aging and is a weak and inconsistent sleep aid. **The Dean's Recommendation: Take melatonin only for jet lag and to reset altered day-night rhythms (see chapter 5).**
✗	Royal jelly	Increases strength, stamina, and longevity Lowers cholesterol Acts as an antioxidant Stimulates the immune system Heals wounds	Royal jelly is made by bees, and honey and bee products do have natural antioxidant properties. Though royal jelly has been found to lower blood cholesterol levels, it's also caused allergic reactions, asthma, and death. **The Dean's Recommendation: Don't take royal jelly.**
✗	Testosterone	Increases libido, muscle strength, and bone density Makes you feel younger	In most men, testosterone levels do decline somewhat with age. However, replacing testosterone has only modest effects in older men with low levels. Men with normal testosterone levels should not take supplemental injections because they increase the risk of prostate enlargement and prostate cancer. **The Dean's Recommendation: Hold off on testosterone until we have more information that the benefits outweigh the risks of prostate disease (see chapter 7).**

Choosing the Best Products

There are many ways to buy supplements; in fact, these days someone seems to be hawking pills everywhere you turn. There are stores that sell nothing but supplements, exclusive spas with proprietary formulas, vast arrays of exotic products on the shelves of health food stores, Web sites making extravagant claims, and new sections springing up at the supermarket to tempt you to skip the fish and veggies and buy some pills and cookies instead.

My recommendation is to get the most bang for your buck by buying

supplements at a chain drug or discount store. Here are a few tips to
keep in mind:

- ⑥ **Cost does not equal quality.** The cost of supplements can vary
  quite widely, but there's no evidence that more expensive
  brands are more potent, soluble, or otherwise good for you. I've
  seen bottles containing the same amount of vitamin E retailing
  from $3.99 to $21.99. The main difference between the products is the $18 missing from your wallet in the latter case.
- ⑥ **Don't trust potency claims.** Supplement makers can get quite
  creative when labeling their products. "Laboratory tested." "Potency guaranteed," they reassure you. But without governing
  regulations, these claims have no particular meaning. It's an
  unfortunate fact that the potency of supplements often fails to
  match what's listed on the label, and we don't have laws in
  place to do anything about it. To make matters worse, many
  supplements aren't formulated to fully dissolve in your intestinal tract, which means you flush the rest away.
- ⑥ **USP means some quality control.** You can gain some quality control assurance by looking for supplements labeled "USP." This indicates approval by the U.S. Pharmacopeia, a nonprofit organization
  that tests supplements for quality and such things as solubility.
- ⑥ **Get the right dose.** Supplements come in many potencies. Be
  sure to take the amount you need, no more or less. The What
  Works shopping list on pages 228–229 provides my recommendations for specific nutritional supplements.

Mirror, Mirror: Shopping for Younger Skin

How do you feel about the skin you're in? You may have the heart and
soul of an 18-year-old, but the first thing other people see is your epi-
dermis, and chances are that if you've been around for a while, it's
showing some signs of age.

Though the medical profession focuses on the health of your inner
systems, how you look affects your self-esteem and how others treat you,
so looking your best is absolutely part of an AgeLess lifestyle. This doesn't
mean I endorse *unproven* cosmetic treatments or excessive investments
of money or time, but you don't have to be vain to be concerned about
the health of your skin. After all, it's the largest organ of your body!

Skin and the Aging Process

Your skin undergoes several changes with age, most of them related to accumulated exposure to the sun. To see how all the rays you've caught have aged your skin, compare a spot that gets plenty of sun—say, your forearm—with an area that never sees the light of day (you choose). Do you see more wrinkling, discoloration, and gray hairs on the exposed skin? That's the sun at work.

Age also causes your skin to lose elasticity, collagen, and underlying fat, all of which can result in wrinkles. If you're a very expressive person, years of scrunching your brow and smiling have also probably cast lines in your face that eventually deepen into wrinkles. Gravity doesn't help matters either; this natural force accounts for your skin's tendency to sag over time. And then there are your genes. Fair-skinned people are more susceptible to skin changes from age and sun exposure than are those with darker skin. Finally, smoking accelerates the rate of age-related changes to skin. Yet another excellent reason to kick the habit.

The chart on the next page outlines common age-related skin conditions.

The New Rules for AgeLess Skin

There are two ways to help your skin age less: prevention and treatment. Obviously prevention is preferable, but sooner or later all skin will start to show its age. Don't panic. You have options.

Preventing skin aging. If you do only one thing to prevent premature aging of the skin, do this: Protect yourself from that big old star that is our source of light and energy on earth, the sun. Like all natural forces, the sun is both beneficent and destructive. It must be treated with respect. Here's how to avoid its wrath.

- **Limit.** Try to stay out of the sun during times of the most intense rays—10:00 A.M. to 4:00 P.M. year-round and most daylight hours during the summer.
- **Protect.** When out in the sun, wear sunscreen with a sun protection factor (SPF) of 15 or higher. Don't forget to protect your eyes by wearing sunglasses. This can help prevent both cataracts and crow's feet. If you'll be out long, opt for protective clothing and wear a wide-brimmed hat.
- **Don't tan.** Sunbathing, going to tanning salons, and using sun-

How to Counter Age-Related Skin Changes

Time, sun exposure, and your habits can cause changes to your skin as you age. Here are some of the most common changes and what you can do to counter them.

Age-Related Change	Description	Tips
Wrinkles	Caused by loss of elasticity in the skin, gravity, sun damage, facial expressions.	For prevention, avoid long periods of sun exposure and use sunscreens (at least SPF 15) and moisturizing creams daily and at night. Treat with Botox, collagen injections, resurfacing, or plastic surgery.
Age (or liver) spots	Flat, brown areas with rounded edges frequently found on the hands, face, back, and feet.	Can be treated with hydroquinone bleach, cryosurgery, or lasers.
Seborrhic keratosis	Raised plaquelike spots.	Sometimes confused with melanoma, so must be seen by a dermatologist. Can be removed with liquid nitrogen.
Spider veins (telangectasias)	Small blood vessels radiating out from a central vessel.	Laser removal is effective in most cases.
Cherry angiomas	Small, bright red, raised rounded spots; actually dilated blood vessels.	Laser removal is quite effective.
Skin cancers	Basal cell carcinoma: The most common type; the cancer cells usually don't metastasize and are easily removed Squamous cell carcinoma: Can invade adjacent tissue but don't usually metastasize Melanoma: The most deadly form of skin cancer, melanoma must be detected and removed early to prevent metastasis.	Limit sun exposure and use high-SPF sunscreen. Early detection and removal are key, so have regular skin checks.
Pruritus (itching)	Age-related loss of lubricating glands leads to dry skin, which can become itchy.	Normal itchy skin can be treated effectively by avoiding hot water and using moisturizing creams. Consult your doctor if you have severe itching that doesn't respond to moisturizing cream, since it may be associated with serious illnesses.
Dandruff	Patches of flaky skin common on scalp, forehead, eyebrows, ears, groin, and chest.	Responds to topical steroid creams, lotions, and solutions, as well as shampoos containing salicylic acid, zinc pyrithione, or tar.

lamps are no-nos. If you like bronze skin, use sunless tanning lotions instead. The products available today are formulated to go on smoothly and evenly; they're much improved over their predecessors. Do get the small amount of daily sun exposure you need for good sleep and synthesis of vitamin D. Chapters 2 and 5 can tell you more about a healthy relationship with the sun.

Taking care of aging skin. The treatment of aging skin is a multibillion-dollar business. The cosmetic companies have been quick to capitalize on our fears of looking older, and the products that line store shelves present literally thousands of variations on their therapeutic claims. My dermatologist friends tell me that most antiaging creams are just souped-up moisturizers. Their net production price per jar? Perhaps a dollar or two. Retail price? The sky's the limit.

The good news is that today there are better treatments available. During the last decade, a number of products have come onto the market that actually make skin look younger. See "Treatments for AgeLess Skin" on the next page for an overview of skin treatment options. Here are some that I recommend:

Topical treatments. The first topical treatment was Retin-A (tretinoin), which works by stimulating the growth of dermal collagen. In the process it also makes skin more sensitive to the sun, so you need to protect your face with sunscreen. Soon after Retin-A came alpha hydroxy acids, which remove the outermost layer of skin cells. Vitamin C and E creams have been found to have modest effects on sun-damaged skin. Kinetin improves the look of skin without the redness and irritation that Retin-A and alpha hydroxy acids can bring.

Injections. For considerably more money and longer-lasting results, you can subject yourself to the needle. Injections of cow collagen, human tissue extracts, or synthetic substances directly into wrinkles can plump them up for somewhere around 6 months, when you'll need another shot to maintain the effect. Synthetic and human materials are preferred, since some people are allergic to cow collagen.

One of the most popular injections is Botox, a powerful poison that works by paralyzing nerves. An experienced dermatologist can inject Botox into a wrinkled area to relax the underlying facial muscles, which temporarily makes the wrinkles disappear. Botox is especially effective for treating wrinkles related to facial expression. Botox is not without

The Lunchtime Peel

Looking for a quick skin lift? You can get a very mild chemical peel that only takes an hour. Some people do it on their lunch hour, then go right back to work. As with other resurfacing treatments, you must keep treated skin moisturized and out of the sun during recovery. Repeat at weekly to monthly intervals.

risks, however. There's a possible danger of temporarily paralyzing muscles around the eyes and mouth, and some users complain that their faces become less expressive after a Botox treatment. As with other injections, you'll need a Botox booster shot about every 6 months.

Resurfacing treatments. Next up the scale of cost and commitment are treatments that resurface the skin. There are several techniques to

Treatments for AgeLess Skin

There are various treatments to give skin a more youthful appearance, including topical treatments, injections, resurfacing, and surgery. I don't recommend hormone replacement therapy as a skin treatment.

Treatment	How quickly it works	How long it lasts
Moisturizing creams	Immediately	As long as applied
Vitamins C and E creams	3 months	As long as applied
Retin-A (Renova)	3 months	As long as applied
Kinetin	3 months	As long as applied
Alpha hydroxy acids	6 months	As long as applied
Collagen, synthetic, and human tissue injections	Immediately	6 months
Botox injections	Immediately	6 months
Chemical peels	1–2 months	1–5 years
Dermabrasion	1–2 months	1–5 years
Laser resurfacing	1–3 months	1–5 years
Plastic surgery	1–2 months	5 or more years
Estrogen replacement	2–3 months	As long as estrogen used

accomplish this. Dermabrasion uses a high-speed rotating brush to re-move the top layers of skin. Chemical peels dissolve the outer skin layers with acids. Peels are generally gentler and less painful than many lasers, which are another resurfacing alternative. All resurfacing techniques can be painful. The exposed skin is swollen and red and recovery usu-ally takes weeks, during which time you'll probably want to keep a low profile and stay out of the sun. During recovery, you'll have to mois-turize your skin continuously to keep it from drying out. When the skin grows back, it has more collagen and looks younger and lighter in color. The good news is that resurfacing lasts for several years. All three resur-facing techniques carry the risks of scarring and skin infection.

Plastic surgery. The most costly and time-consuming type of skin treatment is plastic surgery. But this doesn't keep it from being one of the

Effectiveness (scale of 1 to 4)	Concerns
+	None
+	None
++	Can cause skin redness and irritation and sun sensitivity
++	Fewer side effects than Retin-A or alpha hydroxy acids
++	Can cause skin redness and irritation and sun sensitivity
+++	Collagen made from cow tissue can cause allergic reactions
+++	Loss of some facial expression. Potential small risk of temporary paralysis of certain facial muscles
+++	Painful and costly
+++	Painful and costly
+++	Painful, costly, and long recovery time
++++	Painful and very costly
++	Risks of taking estrogen (see chapter 7)

most common surgical procedures performed in America—and it's not just for women anymore. While during the 1970s, 90 percent of face-lift patients were women, more and more men are taking advantage of this technology. In Los Angeles, my plastic surgeon colleagues estimate that half their patients are men.

A face-lift removes wrinkles and enhances facial tone by literally pulling the skin tighter. The results can last for many years. However, recovery can take weeks, and as with any surgery, there are greater risks than for less invasive procedures. These include infection, bleeding, and scarring, as well as the risks of anesthesia.

Hormones: Not recommended. For women during and after menopause, one benefit of estrogen replacement therapy is its ability to help maintain youthful-looking skin. However, estrogen replacement comes with many risks detailed in chapter 7, and I don't recommend it for this purpose.

There are thousands of longevity products available, with more in the pipeline every day. Most of the price you pay for products and treatments goes to advertising, so don't equate expense with quality. Instead, remember that people have been selling the fountain of youth for centuries. Dismiss flamboyant claims to reverse aging and make well-informed decisions about how to spend your time and money. Most importantly, follow the New Rules and most of your shopping for longevity will already be done.

CHAPTER 9

THE DEAN'S CONCLUDING THOUGHTS

WE CAN TAKE CONTROL OF OUR AGING, but to realize the full potential of this book, you have to begin *today*. Not tomorrow, or the next day, or the next. Most of us have a natural tendency to procrastinate. Sure, you can make excuses and put it off—until that massive heart attack or cancer diagnosis scares you to your senses.

Aging less is a lifetime affair. Here is my suggested game plan for getting started now.

1. **Enlist the support of your spouse, significant other, or friend.** Making lifestyle changes is never easy—even rewarding ones like those I've described in these pages. Sharing the journey with someone close can make the difference between sticking to your goals and quitting when the going gets rough. Give your designated partner a copy of this book and map your AgeLess game plan together.

2. **Take it one New Rule at a time.** Don't let aging less become an overwhelming project. Letting yourself feel stressed over small lapses or not making faster progress could have the opposite effect. Instead take one rule at a time, on your own schedule and at an easy pace. If you usually take a break from your workday at 3 in the afternoon, get in 10 minutes of brisk walking or stretching. If a stop at Starbucks is part of your morning routine, choose a whole grain muffin instead of a white-flour bagel. Use the AgeLess Agendas at the end of the chapters to keep

track of your healthy choices. Charting your progress is another way to keep motivation high.

3. **Start with exercise.** Of all the factors that influence your health and longevity, exercise is the most important. There's no faster way to improve your risk profile for the main causes of death and disability in old age—heart disease, cancer, diabetes, hypertension, obesity, osteoporosis, and memory loss—than to get off the couch. Exercise helps with all the other New Rules, too. If you need to get a good night's sleep or to lose a few pounds, aerobic exercise and weight training will help you reach these goals. Exercise will also improve your mood to give you a head start toward the engagement-related rules, and it works with the healthy diet outlined in the nutrition chapter to maximize your energy every day.

The Future of Aging Less

For anyone committed to aging less, the future looks very exciting. Scientific progress in the field is accelerating rapidly. The Human Genome Project is one of the great scientific feats of all time. This international research effort to sequence and map all human genes will be finished in 2003. However, this is not the end of our quest to understand human disease, but the beginning. Now the second stage begins, in which we identify how these genes and their variations increase or decrease our susceptibility to disease and how they affect the aging processes.

New discoveries in genetics could profoundly change how we prevent and treat heart disease, stroke, type 2 diabetes, Alzheimer's disease, osteoporosis, arthritis, and many cancers. Nanotechnology may even make it possible to change bad genes into good ones, thus reducing our chances of getting a wide variety of diseases tied to genetic susceptibility.

These advances will be accompanied by astonishing progress in bioengineering. We're already in an era in which noninvasive coronary bypass surgery is now possible without opening the patient's chest. Soon, artificial joint replacement will be refined to a point that almost every joint in the human body can be replaced by parts that function even better than the originals.

Artificial eyes and ears will make blindness and deafness obsolete. Stem cell technology will advance to the point that you can use your own cells to generate customized artificial hearts, kidneys, livers, lungs . . . just about any organ, created from your genetic code.

Is it worth making sure you'll still be around to witness all these advances? You better believe it! The average baby boomer who chooses to age less will live into his or her late eighties. By that time, most of these techniques will be available as outpatient procedures in your local neighborhoods.

Your task is to make it to that point, to escape the ravages of age so you can extend vital youthfulness in the present, and to avail yourself of powerful longevity technologies in the future. The New Rules can help get you there—and to your hundredth birthday—*if* you start today.

Foods That Extend Your Healthspan

Food glorious food—when it comes to AgeLess living, there's no better source of most nutrients you need. To help you keep track of your daily intake, here are some of the best, grouped according to the AgeLess nutrients they richly contain.

Vitamin C

Below are some of the foods high in vitamin C. Put these on your grocery list:

Food Source	Serving Size	Vitamin C Content (mg)
Peppers, sweet, red, raw	1 pepper	226
Papayas, raw	1 papaya	188
Peppers, hot chile, red or green, raw	1 pepper	109
Peppers, sweet, green, raw	1 pepper	106
Orange juice, fresh	6 oz	93
General Mills' Total cereal	1 cup	80
Kiwifruit, fresh, raw	1 medium	75
Orange juice, from frozen concentrate	6 oz	73
Grapefruit juice, pink	6 oz	70
Oranges, raw	1 orange	70
Cranberry juice cocktail, bottled	6 oz	67
Broccoli, boiled, drained	½ cup	58
Mangos, raw	1 mango	57
Soup, tomato, canned, prepared with equal volume water	6 oz	50
Vegetable juice cocktail, canned	6 oz	50

Food Source	Serving Size	Vitamin C Content (mg)
Brussels sprouts, boiled, drained	½ cup	48
Chestnuts, European, roasted	1 oz	47
Strawberries, raw	½ cup	47
General Mills' Total Corn Flakes cereal	1 cup	45
Broccoli, raw	½ cup	41

Source: U.S. Department of Agriculture, Agricultural Research Service. 2001. USDA National Nutrient Database for Standard Reference, Release 14. Nutrient Data Laboratory, http://www.nal.usda.gov/fnic/foodcomp

Carotenoids

Following are some of the foods with the highest carotenoid counts:

Food (100-g/3 ½-oz edible portion)	Total Carotenoids (mcg)
Kale, raw	48,776
Tomato paste, canned	30,771
Kale, boiled	22,000
Carrots, frozen, boiled	17,814
Ketchup	17,738
Spinach, raw	17,535
Pureed tomatoes, canned	17,170
Pasta sauce, spaghetti/marinara, ready-to-serve	16,590
Tomato sauce, canned	16,327
Mangos, canned, drained	14,670
Carrots, raw	13,485
Turnip greens, boiled	13,015
Collards, boiled, drained	12,619
Spinach, boiled, drained	12,285
Carrots, boiled, drained	12,124
Carrots, baby, raw	12,058
Pumpkin, canned	11,735
Tomato soup, canned, condensed	11,245

(continued)

Carotenoids (cont.)

Food (100-g/3 ½-oz edible portion)	Total Carotenoids (mcg)
Vegetable juice cocktail, canned	10,780
Tomatoes, red, ripe, canned	9,934
Tomato juice, canned	9,806
Sweet potato, cooked, baked in skin, without salt	9,488
Carrots, canned, drained	9,246
Sweet potato, canned, vacuum pack	8,314
Apricots, canned, heavy syrup, drained	6,705
Squash, winter, butternut, baked	5,700
Watermelon, raw	5,283
Spinach, canned, drained	4,820
Peppers, sweet, red, raw	4,643
Vegetarian vegetable soup, canned, condensed	4,000
Lettuce, cos or romaine, raw	3,907
Tomatoes, red, ripe, raw	3,660
Beet greens, raw	3,410
Broccoli, boiled	3,268
Broccoli, raw	3,225
Beef stew with vegetables (including potatoes and carrots), canned	2,842
Minestrone soup, canned, condensed	2,760
Vegetable beef soup, canned, condensed	2,563
Beet greens, boiled	2,560
Apricots, raw	2,559
Grapefruit, pink and red, raw	2,095

Source: USDA-NCC Carotenoid Database for U.S. Foods—1998

Fiber

To add more fiber to your diet, choose the following sources of this health-protecting, appetite-controlling nutrient:

Food Source	Serving Size	Fiber Content (g)
Kellogg's All-Bran cereal	1 cup	19.38
Kidney beans, red, canned	1 cup	16.38
Prunes, dried, stewed	1 cup	16.37
Peas, split, boiled	1 cup	16.27
Lentils, boiled	1 cup	15.64
Black beans, boiled	1 cup	14.96
Pinto beans, boiled	1 cup	14.71
Oat bran, raw	1 cup	14.48
Refried beans, canned	1 cup	13.36
Dates, dry	1 cup	13.35
Lima beans, boiled	1 cup	13.16
Kidney beans, red, boiled	1 cup	13.10
Beans, baked, plain or vegetarian, canned	1 cup	12.70
Chickpeas (garbanzo beans), boiled	1 cup	12.46
Navy beans, boiled	1 cup	11.65
Lima beans, canned	1 cup	11.57
Black-eyed peas, boiled	1 cup	11.18
Raspberries, red, frozen	1 cup	11.00
Lima beans, baby, frozen, boiled	1 cup	10.80
Tomato products, paste, canned	1 cup	10.74
Chickpeas (garbanzo beans), canned	1 cup	10.56
Soybeans, boiled	1 cup	10.32
Pears, Asian, raw	1 pear	9.90

(continued)

Fiber (cont.)

Food Source	Serving Size	Fiber Content (g)
Artichokes, globe or french, boiled	1 cup	9.07
Peas, green, frozen, boiled	1 cup	8.91
Raspberries, raw	1 cup	8.36
Kellogg's Raisin Bran cereal	1 cup	8.17

Source: U.S. Department of Agriculture, Agricultural Research Service. 2001. USDA National Nutrient Database for Standard Reference, Release 14. Nutrient Data Laboratory, http://www.nal.usda.gov/fnic/foodcomp

Calcium

By and large, dairy products are some of the best sources of calcium, but plenty of nondairy alternatives exist—see below:

Food Source	Serving Size	Calcium Content (mg)
Yogurt, plain, fat-free	8-oz container	452
Yogurt, plain, low-fat	8-oz container	415
Yogurt, fruit, low-fat	8-oz container	345
General Mills' Total cereal	1 cup	344
Sardines, Atlantic, canned in oil, drained solids with bone	3 oz	325
General Mills' Basic 4 cereal	1 cup	310
Milk, fat-free or low-fat	1 cup	301
Milk, 2% milkfat	1 cup	298
Swiss cheese	1 oz	272
General Mills' Total Raisin Bran cereal	1 cup	238
Provolone cheese	1 oz	214
Kellogg's All-Bran cereal	1 cup	212
Mozzarella cheese, part-skim milk, low-moisture	1 oz	207

Food Source	Serving Size	Calcium Content (mg)
Cheddar cheese	1 oz	204
Muenster cheese	1 oz	203
General Mills' Total Corn Flakes cereal	1 cup	178
American cheese, pasteurized	1 oz	175
Instant oatmeal, fortified, plain, prepared with water	1 packet	163
Feta cheese	1 oz	140
General Mills' Honey Nut Chex cereal	1 cup	136
Quaker Cinnamon Life cereal	1 cup	135
Soybeans, green, cooked, boiled, drained	½ cup	131
Tofu, firm, prepared with calcium sulfate and magnesium chloride (nigari)	¼ block	131
Cheddar cheese, low-fat	1 oz	118
Colby cheese, low-fat	1 oz	118
Ocean perch, Atlantic, cooked	3 oz	116
Collards, cooked, drained	½ cup	113
Ice cream, French vanilla, soft-serve	½ cup	113
Black-eyed peas, cooked, boiled, drained, without salt	½ cup	106
Quaker instant oatmeal, prepared with water	1 packet	105
General Mills' Corn Chex cereal	1 cup	100
English muffins, plain, enriched (includes sourdough)	1 muffin	99
Quaker Life cereal, plain	¾ cup	98
Cocoa mix powder, without added nutrients, prepared with water	1 serving	97
Blue crab, cooked	3 oz	88
Soybeans, mature, boiled	½ cup	88
Cheese, ricotta, part-skim milk	1 oz	84

(continued)

Calcium (*cont.*)

Food Source	Serving Size	Calcium Content (mg)
Ice cream, vanilla	½ cup	84
General Mills' Rice Chex cereal	1 cup	83
Cabbage, Chinese (bok choy), boiled, drained	½ cup	79
General Mills' Raisin Nut Bran cereal	1 cup	74
Papayas, raw	1 papaya	73
Rainbow trout, farmed, cooked	3 oz	73
General Mills' Honey Nut Clusters cereal	1 cup	72
Almonds	1 oz (24 nuts)	70
Parmesan cheese, grated	1 tablespoon	69
Bagels, plain, enriched, with calcium propionate (includes onion, poppy, sesame)	4" bagel	66
Herring, Atlantic, pickled	3 oz	65
Baked beans, plain or vegetarian, canned	½ cup	64
Navy beans, boiled	½ cup	64
Crab cakes, blue crab	1 cake	63
Haddock, cooked	1 fillet	63
General Mills' Wheat Chex cereal	1 cup	60
Figs, dried, uncooked	2 figs	55
General Mills' Cheerios cereal	1 cup	55
General Mills' Wheaties cereal	1 cup	55
Artichokes, globe or french, boiled, drained	1 medium	54
Lobster, northern, cooked	3 oz	52
Mustard greens, boiled, drained	½ cup	52
Oranges, raw	1 orange	52

Food Source	Serving Size	Calcium Content (mg)
Halibut, Atlantic and Pacific, cooked	3 oz	51
Okra, boiled, drained	½ cup	51
Alaskan king crab, cooked	3 oz	50
Brazil nuts, dried, unblanched	1 oz (6–8 nuts)	50
Cream of Wheat cereal, regular or quick, cooked with water	1 cup	50
Shrimp, canned	3 oz	50

Source: U.S. Department of Agriculture, Agricultural Research Service. 2001. USDA National Nutrient Database for Standard Reference, Release 14. Nutrient Data Laboratory, http://www.nal.usda.gov/fnic/foodcomp

Vitamin E

Sources of this beneficial antioxidant include the following:

Food Source	Serving Size	Vitamin E Content (IU)
Sunflower seed kernels, dry roasted	¼ cup	16.1
Tomato paste, canned	1 cup	11.3
Almonds	1 oz (24 nuts)	7.4
Sunflower oil, linoleic	1 tablespoon	6.9
Pureed tomatoes, canned	1 cup	6.3
Safflower oil, salad or cooking, oleic	1 tablespoon	4.7
Hazelnuts or filberts	1 oz (20 nuts)	4.3
Oil, soybean, salad or cooking	1 tablespoon	3.8
Papayas, raw	1 papaya	3.4
Soybeans, boiled	1 cup	3.4

Source: U.S. Department of Agriculture, Agricultural Research Service. 2001. USDA National Nutrient Database for Standard Reference, Release 14. Nutrient Data Laboratory, http://www.nal.usda.gov/fnic/foodcomp

Folate

To get more folate in your diet, look to the following sources of this vitamin:

Food Source	Serving Size	Folate Content (mcg)
General Mills' Total cereal	1 cup	901
General Mills' Wheat Chex cereal	1 cup	407
General Mills' Cheerios	1 cup	336
General Mills' Kix	1 cup	252
Quaker Life cereal	1 cup	237
Kellogg's Smacks cereal	1 cup	222
Kellogg's Raisin Bran cereal	1 cup	199
Black-eyed peas, boiled	½ cup	179
Lentils, boiled	½ cup	179
Turnip greens, boiled, drained	1 cup	170
Egg noodles, enriched, cooked	1 cup	166
General Mills' Wheaties cereal	1 cup	166
Kellogg's Corn Flakes cereal	1 cup	164
Kellogg's Rice Krispies cereal	1 cup	158
Kellogg's Special K cereal	1 cup	154
Pinto beans, boiled	½ cup	147
Chickpeas (garbanzo beans), boiled	½ cup	141
Spinach, boiled, drained	½ cup	131
Black beans, boiled	½ cup	128
Navy beans, boiled	½ cup	127
Papayas, raw	1 papaya	116
Kidney beans, boiled	½ cup	115
Soybeans, green, boiled, drained	½ cup	100
Asparagus, boiled, drained	4 spears	88
Collards, boiled, drained	½ cup	88

Food Source	Serving Size	Folate Content (mcg)
Orange juice, from frozen concentrate	6 oz	82
Lettuce, cos or romaine, raw	1 cup	78
Rice, white, long-grain, cooked	½ cup	77
Beets, boiled, drained	½ cup	68
Kidney beans, red, canned	½ cup	65
Peas, boiled	½ cup	64
Lima beans, large, canned	½ cup	60
Spinach, raw	1 cup	58
Oranges, raw	1 cup	54
Mustard greens, boiled, drained	½ cup	51

Source: U.S. Department of Agriculture, Agricultural Research Service. 2001. USDA National Nutrient Database for Standard Reference, Release 14. Nutrient Data Laboratory, http://www.nal.usda.gov/fnic/foodcomp

Select References

Chapter 1

Rowe, J. W. and Kahn, R. L. *Successful Aging*. (1998). New York: Pantheon Books.

Chapter 2

General

Balluz, L. S., Kieszak, S. M., Philen, R., and Mulinare, J. "Vitamin and Mineral Supplement Use in the United States: Results from the Third National Health and Nutrition Examination Survey." *Archives of Family Medicine* 9 (2000): 258–62.

De Lorgeril, M., Salen, P., Martin, J-L., Monjaud, I., Delaye, J., and Mamelle, N. "Mediterranean Diet, Traditional Risk Factors, and the Rate of Cardiovascular Complications after Myocardial Infarction: Final Report of the Lyon Diet Heart Study." *Circulation* 99 (1999): 779–85.

Frazao, E. "America's Eating Habits: Changes and Consequences." Economic Research Service *Agriculture Information Bulletin* 750 (1999): 5–32.

Kouris-Blazos, A., Gnardellis, C., Wahlqvist, M. L., Trichopoulos, D., Lukito, W., and Trichopoulou, A. "Are the Advantages of the Mediterranean Diet Transferable to Other Populations? A Cohort Study in Melbourne, Australia." *British Journal of Nutrition* 82 (1999): 57–61.

Krauss, R. M., Eckel, R. H., Howard, B., Appel, L. J., Daniels, S. R., Deckelbaum, R. J., Erdman, J. W., Kris-Etherton, P., Goldberg, I. J., Kotchen, T. A., Lichtenstein, A. H., Mitch, W. E., Mullis, R., Robinson, K., Wylie-Rosett, J., St. Jeor, S., Suttie, J., Tribble, D. L., and Bazzarre, T. L. "Revision 2000: A Statement for

Healthcare Professionals from the Nutrition Committee of the American Heart Association." *Journal of Nutrition* 131 (2001): 132–46.

Kris-Etherton, P., Eckel, R. H., Howard, B. V., St. Jeor, S., and Bazzarre, T. L. "Lyon Diet Heart Study: Benefits of a Mediterranean-Style, National Cholesterol Education Program/American Heart Association Step I Dietary Pattern on Cardiovascular Disease." *Circulation* 103 (2001): 1823–25.

Alcohol

Berger, K. B., Ajani, U. A., Kase, C. S., Gaziano, J. M., Buring, J. E., Glynn, R. J., and Hennekens, C. H. "Light-to-Moderate Alcohol Consumption and the Risk of Stroke Among U.S. Male Physicians." *New England Journal of Medicine* 341 (1999): 1557–64.

Goldberg, I. J., Mosca, L., Piano, M. R., and Fisher, E. A. "Wine and Your Heart: A Science Advisory for Healthcare Professionals from the Nutrition Committee, Council on Epidemiology and Prevention, and Council on Cardiovascular Nursing of the American Heart Association." *Stroke* 103 (2001): 591–94.

Hommel, M., and Jaillar, A. "Alcohol for Stroke Prevention?" *New England Journal of Medicine* 341 (1999): 1605–6.

Potter, J. D. "Hazards and Benefits of Alcohol." *New England Journal of Medicine* 337 (1997): 1763–64.

Rimm, E. B., Klatsky, A., Grobbee, D., and Stampfer, M. J. "Review of Moderate Alcohol Consumption and Reduced Risk of Coronary Heart Disease: Is the Effect Due to Beer, Wine, or Spirits?" *British Medical Journal* 312 (1996): 731–36.

Rimm, E. B., Williams, P., Fosher, K., Criqui, M., and Stampfer, M. J. "Moderate Alcohol Intake and Lower Risk of Coronary Heart Disease: Meta-Analysis of Effects on Lipids and Haemostatic Factors." *British Medical Journal* 319 (1999): 1523–28.

Shaper, A. G., and Wannamethee, S. G. "Alcohol Intake and Mortality in Middle Aged Men with Diagnosed Coronary Heart Disease." *Heart* 83 (2000): 394–99.

Thun, M. J., Peto, R., Lopez, A. D., Monaco, J. H., Henley, S. J., Hearth, C. W., and Doll, R. "Alcohol Consumption and Mortality Among Middle-Aged and Elderly U.S. Adults." *New England Journal of Medicine* 337 (1997): 1705–14.

Wannamethee, S. G., and Shaper, A. G. "Taking Up Regular Drinking in Middle Age: Effect on Major Coronary Heart Disease Events and Mortality." *Heart* 87 (2002): 32–36.

Antioxidants/Carotenoids

Arab, L., and Steck, S. "Lycopene and Cardiovascular Disease." *American Journal of Clinical Nutrition* 71 (2000): 1691S–95S.

Block, G., Norkus, E., Hudes, M., Mandel, S., and Helzlsouer, K. "Which Plasma Antioxidants Are Most Related to Fruit and Vegetable Consumption?" *American Journal of Epidemiology* 154 (2001): 1113–18.

Brown, B. G., Zhao, X-Q., Chait, A., Fisher, L. D., Cheung, M. C., Morse, J. S., Dowdy, A. A., Marino, E. K., Bolson, E. L., Alaupovic, P., Frohlich, J., and Albers, J. J. "Simvastatin and Niacin, Antioxidant Vitamins, or the Combination for the Prevention of Coronary Disease." *New England Journal of Medicine* 345 (2001): 1583–92.

Cramer, D. W., Kuper, H., Harlow, B. L., and Titus-Ernstoff, L. "Carotenoids, Antioxidants and Ovarian Cancer Risk in Pre- and Postmenopausal Women." *International Journal of Cancer* 94 (2001): 128–34.

Cummings, J. H., and Bingham, S. A. "Diet and the Prevention of Cancer." *British Medical Journal* 317 (1998): 1636–40.

Diaz, M. N., Frei, B., Vita, J. A., and Keaney, J. F. "Antioxidants and Atherosclerotic Heart Disease." *New England Journal of Medicine* 337 (1997): 408–16.

Freedman, J. E. "Antioxidant Versus Lipid-Altering Therapy—Some Answers, More Questions." *New England Journal of Medicine* 345 (2001): 1636–37.

Gaziano, J. M., Manson, J. E., Branch, L. G., Colditz, G. A., Willett, W. C., and Buring, J. E. "A Prospective Study of Consumption of Carotenoids in Fruits and Vegetables and Decreased Cardiovascular Mortality in the Elderly." *Annals of Epidemiology* 5 (1995): 255–60.

Hennekens, C. H., Buring, J. E., Manson, J. E., Stampfer, M., Rosner, B., Cook, N. R., Belanger, C., LaMotte, F., Gaziano, J. M., Ridker, P. M., Willett, W. C., and Peto, R. "Lack of Effect of Long-Term Supplementation with Beta Carotene on the Incidence of Malignant Neoplasms and Cardiovascular Disease." *New England Journal of Medicine* 334 (1996): 1145–49.

Hirvonen, T., Virtamo, J., Korhonen, P., Albanes, D., Pietinen, P. "Intake of Flavonoids, Carotenoids, Vitamins C and E, and Risk of Stroke in Male Smokers." *Stroke* 31 (2000): 2301–6.

Knekt, P., Reunanen, A., Jarvinen, R., Seppanen, R., Heliovaara, M., and Aromaa, A. "Antioxidant Vitamin Intake and Coronary Mortality in a Longitudinal Population Study." *American Journal of Epidemiology* 139 (1994): 1180–9.

Kritchevsky, S. B. "Beta-Carotene, Carotenoids and the Prevention of Coronary Heart Disease." *Journal of Nutrition* 129 (1999): 5–8.

Lee, I.-M., Cook, N. R., Manson, J. E., Buring, J. E., and Hennekens, C. H. "Beta-Carotene Supplementation and Incidence of Cancer and Cardiovascular Disease: The Women's Health Study." *Journal of the National Cancer Institute* 91 (1999): 2102–6.

Michaud, D. S., Feskanich, D., Rimm, E. B., Colditz, G. A., Speizer, F. E., Willett, W. C., and Giovannucci, E. "Intake of Specific Carotenoids and Risk of Lung Cancer in 2 Prospective US Cohorts." *American Journal of Clinical Nutrition* 72 (2000): 990–97.

Tardif, J-C., Gilles Coté, G., Lespérance, J., Bourassa, M., Lambert, J., Doucet, S., Bilodeau, L., Nattel, S., de Guise, P., and Multivitamins and Probucol Study Group. "Probucol and Multivitamins in the Prevention of Restenosis after Coronary Angioplasty." *New England Journal of Medicine* 337 (1997): 365–72.

Tribble, D. L. "Antioxidant Consumption and Risk of Coronary Heart Disease: Emphasis on Vitamin C, Vitamin E, and Beta-Carotene. A Statement for Healthcare Professionals from the American Heart Association." *Circulation* 99 (1999): 591–95.

Willett, W. C., and Stampfer, M. J. "What Vitamins Should I Be Taking, Doctor?" *New England Journal of Medicine* 345 (2001): 1819–24.

Young, I. S., and Woodside, J. V. "Antioxidants in Health and Disease." *Journal of Clinical Pathology* 54 (2001): 176–86.

Zhang, S., Hunter, D. J., Forman, M. R., Rosner, B. A., Speizer, F. E., Colditz, F. A., Manson, J. E., Hankinson, S. E., and Willett, W. C. "Dietary Carotenoids and Vitamins A, C, and E and Risk of Breast Cancer." *Journal of the National Cancer Institute* 91 (1999): 547–56.

Calcium

Baron, J. A., Beach, M., Mandel, J. S., van Stolk, R. U., Haile, R. W., Sandler, R. S., Rothstein, R., Summers, R. W., Snover, D. C., Beck, G. J., Bond, J. H., and Greenberg, E. R. "Calcium Supplements for the Prevention of Colorectal Adenomas." *New England Journal of Medicine* 340 (1999): 101–7.

Peacock, M., Liu, G., Carey, M., McClintock, R., Ambrosius, W., Hui, S., and Johnston, C. C. "Effect of Calcium or 25 (OH) Vitamin D_3 Dietary Supplementation on Bone Loss at the Hip in Men and Women over the Age of 60." *Journal of Clinical Endocrinology and Metabolism* 85 (2000): 3011–19.

Chocolate

Carnesecchi, S., Schneider, Y., Lazarus, S. A., Coehlo, D., Gosse, F., and Raul, F. "Flavonols and Procyanidins of Cocoa and Chocolate Inhibit Growth and Polyamine Biosynthesis of Human Colonic Cancer." *Cancer Letters* 175 (2002): 147–55.

Kris-Etherton, P. M., Derr, J. A., Mustad, V. A., Seligson, F. H., and Pearson, T. A. "Effects of a Milk Chocolate Bar Per Day Substituted for a High-Carbohydrate Snack in Young Men on a NCEP/AHA Step 1 Diet." *American Journal of Clinical Nutrition* 60 (1994): 1037S–42S.

Nestel, P. J. "How Good Is Chocolate?" *American Journal of Clinical Nutrition* 74 (2001): 563–64.

Rein, D., Lotito, S., Holt, R. R., Keen, C. L., Schmitz, H. H., and Fraga, C. G. "Epicatechin in Human Plasma: In Vivo Determination and Effect of Chocolate Consumption on Plasma Oxidation Status." *Journal of Nutrition* 130 (2000): 2109S–14S.

Shahkhalili, Y., Murset, C., Meirim, I., Duruz, E., Guinchard, S., Cavadini, C., and Acheson, K. "Calcium Supplementation of Chocolate: Effect on Cocoa Butter Digestibility and Blood Lipids in Humans." *American Journal of Clinical Nutrition* 73 (2001): 246–52.

Wan, Y., Vinson, J. A., Etherton, T. D., Proch, J., Lazarus, S. A., and Kris-Etherton, P. M. "Effects of Cocoa Powder and Dark Chocolate on LDL Oxidative Susceptibility and Prostaglandin Concentrations in Humans." *American Journal of Clinical Nutrition* 74 (2001): 596–602.

Fiber

Aldoori, W. H., Giovannucci, E. L., Rockett, H. R. H., Sampson, L., Rimm, E. B., and Willett, W. C. "A Prospective Study of Dietary Fiber Types and Symptomatic Diverticular Disease in Men." *The Journal of Nutrition* 128 (1998): 714–19.

Liu, S., Manson, J. E., Stampfer, M. J., Rexrode, K. M., Hu, F. B., Rimm, E. B., and Willett, W. C. "Whole Grain Consumption and Risk of Ischemic Stroke in Women: A Prospective Study." *JAMA* 284 (2000): 1534–40.

Folic Acid

Ames, B. N. "DNA Damage from Micronutrient Deficiencies Is Likely to Be a Major Cause of Cancer." *Mutation Research* 475 (2001): 7–20.

De Bree, A., Verschuren, W. M. M., Blom, H. J., and Kromhout, D. "Association between B Vitamin Intake and Plasma Homocysteine Concentration in the General Dutch Population Aged 20–65 y." *American Journal of Clinical Nutrition* 73 (2001): 1027–33.

Jacques, P. F., Selhub, J., Bostom, A. G., Wilson, P. W. F., and Rosenberg, I. H. "The Effect of Folic Acid Fortification on Plasma Folate and Total Homocysteine Concentrations." *New England Journal of Medicine* 340 (1999): 1449–54.

Schnyder, G., Roffi, M., Pin, R., Flammer, Y., Lange, H., Eberli, F. R., Meier, B., Turi, Z. G., and Hess, O. M. "Decreased Rate of Coronary Restenosis after Lowering of Plasma Homocysteine Levels." *New England Journal of Medicine* 345 (2001): 1593–600.

Verhaar, M. C., Stroes, E., and Rabelink, T. J. "Folates and Cardiovascular Disease." *Arteriosclerosis, Thrombosis, and Vascular Biology* 22 (2002): 6–13.

Voutilainen, S., Rissanen, T. H., Virtanen, J., Lakka, T. A., and Salonen, J. T. "Low Dietary Folate Intake Is Associated with an Excess Incidence of Acute Coronary Events: The Kuopio Ischemic Heart Disease Risk Factor Study." *Circulation* 103 (2001): 2674–80.

Homocysteine

De Bree, A., Verschuren, W. M. M., Blom, H., and Kromhout, D. "Lifestyle Factors and Plasma Homocysteine Concentrations in a General Population Sample." *American Journal of Epidemiology* 154 (2001): 150–54.

Knekt, P., Reunanen, A., Alfthan, G., Heliövaara, M., Rissanen, H., Marniemi, J., and Aromaa, A. "Hyperhomocystinemia: A Risk Factor or a Consequence of Coronary Heart Disease?" *Archives of Internal Medicine* 161 (2001): 1589–94.

Omenn, G. S., Beresford, S. A. A., and Motulsky, A. G. "Preventing Coronary Heart Disease: B Vitamins and Homocysteine." *Circulation* 97 (1998): 421–24.

Verhoef, P., Kok, F. J., Kruyssen, D. A. C. M., Schouten, E. G, Witteman, J. C. M., Grobbee, D. E., Ueland, P. M., and Refsum, H. "Plasma Total Homocysteine, B Vitamins, and Risk of Coronary Atherosclerosis." *Arteriosclerosis, Thrombosis, and Vascular Biology* 17 (1997): 989–95.

Nuts

Fraser, G. E. "Nut Consumption, Lipids, and Risk of a Coronary Event." *Clinical Cardiology* 22 (1999): III11–15.

Hu, F. B., and Stampfer, M. J. "Nut Consumption and Risk of Coronary Heart Disease: A Review of Epidemiologic Evidence." *Current Atherosclerosis Reports* 1 (1999): 204–9.

Kris-Etherton, P. M., Zhao, G., Binkoski, A. E., Coval, S. M., and Etherton, T. D. "The Effects of Nuts on Coronary Heart Disease Risk." *Nutrition Reviews* 59 (2001): 103–11.

Tunstall-Pedoe, H. "Nuts to You (. . . and You, and You): Eating Nuts May Be Beneficial—Though It Is Unclear Why." *British Medical Journal* 317 (1998): 1332–33.

Zambón, D., Sabaté, J., Muñoz, S., Campero, B., Casals, E., Merlos, M., Laguan, J. C., and Ros, E. "Substituting Walnuts for Monounsaturated Fat Improves the Serum Lipid Profile of Hypercholesterolemic Men and Women." *Annals of Internal Medicine* 132 (2000): 538–46.

Omega-3

Bigger, J. T., and El-Sherif, T. "Polyunsaturated Fatty Acids and Cardiovascular Events: A Fish Tale." *Circulation* 103 (2001): 623–25.

Daviglus, M. L., Stamler, J., Orencia, A. J., Dyer, A. R., Liu, K., Greenland, P., Walsh, M. K., Morris, D., and Shekelle, R. B. "Fish Consumption and the 30-Year Risk of Fatal Myocardial Infarction." *New England Journal of Medicine* 336 (1997): 1046–53.

Nestel, P. J. "Fish Oil and Cardiovascular Disease: Lipids and Arterial Function." *American Journal of Clinical Nutrition* 71 (2000): 228–31.

Rissanen, T., Voutilainen, S., Nyyssönen, K., Lakka, T. A., and Salonen, J. T. "Fish Oil-Derived Fatty Acids, Docosahexaenoic Acid and Docosapentaenoic Acid, and the Risk of Acute Coronary Events: The Kuopio Ischaemic Heart Disease Risk Factor Study." *Circulation* 102 (2000): 2677–79.

Vitamin B_{12}

Baik, H. W., and Russell, R. M. "Vitamin B_{12} Deficiency in the Elderly." *Annual Review of Nutrition* 19 (1999): 357–77.

Carmel, R. "Current Concepts in Cobalamin Deficiency." *Annual Review of Medicine* 51 (2000): 357–75.

Kuzminski, A. M., Del Giacco, E. J., Allen, R. H., Stabler, S. P., and Lindenbaum, J. "Effective Treatment of Cobalamin Deficiency with Oral Cobalamin." *Blood* 92 (1998): 1191–98.

Kuzniarz, M., Mitchell, P., Cumming, R. G., and Flood, V. M. "Use of Vitamin Supplements and Cataract: The Blue Mountains Eye Study." *American Journal of Ophthalmology* 132 (2001): 19–26.

Lindenbaum, J., Rosenberg, I. H., Wilson, P. W., Stabler, S. P., and Allen, R. H. "Prevalence of Cobalamin Deficiency in the Framingham Elderly Population." *American Journal of Clinical Nutrition* 60 (1994): 2–11.

Penninx, B. W. J. H., Guralnik, J. M., Ferrucci, L., Fried, L. P., Allen, R. H., and Stabler, S. P. "Vitamin B_{12} Deficiency and Depression in Physically Disabled Older Women: Epidemiologic Evidence from the Women's Health and Aging Study." *American Journal of Psychiatry* 157 (2000): 715–21.

Van Asselt, D. Z., Pasman, J. W., van Lier, H. J., Vingerhoets, D. M., Poels, P. J., Kuin, Y., Blom, H. J., and Hoefnagles, W. H. "Cobalamin Supplementation Improves Cognitive and Cerebral Function in Older, Cobalamin-Deficient Persons." *Journal of Gerontology: Medical Sciences* 56A (2001): M775–79.

Wang, H-X., Whalin, A., Basun, H., Fastbom, J., Winblad, B., and Fratiglioni, L. "Vitamin B_{12} and Folate in Relation to the Development of Alzheimer's Disease." *Neurology* 56 (2001): 1188–94.

Vitamin C

Gey, K. F., Stahelin, H. B., and Eichholzer, M. "Poor Plasma Status of Carotene and Vitamin C Is Associated with Higher Mortality from Ischemic Heart Disease and Stroke: Basel Prospective Study." *Clinical Investigator* 71 (1993): 3–6.

Langlois, M., Duprez, D., Delanghe, J., De Buyzere, M., and Clement, D. L. "Serum Vitamin C Concentration Is Low in Peripheral Arterial Disease and Is Associated with Inflammation and Severity of Atherosclerosis." *Circulation* 103 (2001): 1863–68.

Yokoyama, T., Date, C., Kokubo, Y., Yoshiike, N., Matsumura, Y., and Tanaka, H. "Serum Vitamin C Concentration Was Inversely Associated with Subsequent 20-Year Incidence of Stroke in a Japanese Rural Community: The Shibata Study." *Stroke* 31 (2000): 2287–94.

Vitamin D

Fuleihan, G. E-H., and Deeb, M. "Hypovitaminosis D in a Sunny Country." *New England Journal of Medicine* 340 (1999): 1840–41.

Gennari, C. "Calcium and Vitamin D Nutrition and Bone Disease of the Elderly." *Public Health Nutrition* 4 (2001): 547–59.

Holick, M. F. "Environmental Factors That Influence the Cutaneous Production of Vitamin D." *American Journal of Clinical Nutrition* 61 (1995): 638S–45S.

Mawer, E. B., and Davies, M. "Vitamin D Nutrition and Bone Disease in Adults." *Reviews in Endocrine and Metabolic Disorders* 2 (2001): 153–64.

Utiger, R. D. "The Need for More Vitamin D." *New England Journal of Medicine* 338 (1998): 828–29.

Vieth, R., Chan, P-C. R., and MacFarlane, G. D. "Efficacy and Safety of Vitamin D_3 Intake Exceeding the Lowest Observed Adverse Effect Level." *American Journal of Clinical Nutrition* 73 (2001): 288–94.

Vitamin E

Ascherio, A. "Antioxidants and Stroke." *American Journal of Clinical Nutrition* 72 (2000): 337–38.

Collaborative Group of the Primary Prevention Project. "Low-Dose Aspirin and Vitamin E in People at Cardiovascular Risk: A Randomised Trial in General Practice. Collaborative Group of the Primary Prevention Project." *Lancet* 357 (2001): 89–95.

Kaul, N., Devaraj, S., and Jialal, I. "[alpha]-Tocopherol and Atherosclerosis." *Experimental Biology and Medicine* 226 (2001): 5–12.

Keith, M. E., Jeejeebhoy, K. N., Langer, A., Kurian, R., Barr, A., O'Kelly, B., and Sole, M. J. "A Controlled Clinical Trial of Vitamin E Supplementation in Patients with Congestive Heart Failure." *American Journal of Clinical Nutrition* 73 (2001): 219–24.

Lonn, E. M., Yusuf, S., Dzavik, V., Doris, C. I., Yi, Q., Smith, S., Moore-Cox, A., Bosch, J., Riley, W. A., Teo, K. K., and SECURE Investigators. "Effects of Ramipril and Vitamin E on Atherosclerosis: The Study to Evaluate Carotid Ultrasound Changes in Patients Treated with Ramipril and Vitamin E (SECURE)." *Circulation* 103 (2001): 919–25.

Rimm, E. B., Stampfer, M. J., Ascherio, A., Giovannucci. E., Colditz, G. A., Willett, W. C. "Vitamin E Consumption and the Risk of Coronary Disease in Men." *New England Journal of Medicine* 328 (1993): 1450–56.

Stampfer, M. J., Hennekens, C. H , Manson, J. E., Colditz, G. A., Rosner, B., Willett, W. C. "Vitamin E Consumption and the Risk of Coronary Disease in Women." *New England Journal of Medicine* 328 (1993): 1444–49.

Yochum, L. A., Folsom, A. R., and Kushi, L. H. "Intake of Antioxidant Vitamins and Risk of Death from Stroke in Postmenopausal Women." *American Journal of Clinical Nutrition* 72 (2000): 476–83.

Yusuf, S., Dagenais, G., Pogue, J., Bosch, J., and Sleight, P. "Vitamin E Supplementation and Cardiovascular Events in High-Risk Patients. The Heart Outcomes Prevention Evaluation Study Investigators." *New England Journal of Medicine* 342 (2000): 154–60.

No authors listed. "MRC/BHF Heart Protection Study of Antioxidant Vitamin Supplementation in 20,536 High-Risk Individuals: A Randomised Placebo-Controlled Trial." *Lancet* 360 (2002): 23–33.

Chapter 3

Exercise and Age

Christmas, C., and Andersen, R. A. "Exercise and Older Patients: Guidelines for the Clinician." *Journal of the American Geriatrics Society* 48 (2000): 318–24.

Jette, A. M., Lachman, M., Giorgetti, M. M., Assmann, S. F., Harris, B. A., Levenson, C., Wernick, M., and Krebs, D. "Exercise: It's Never Too Late: The Strong-for-Life Program." *American Journal of Public Health* 89 (1999): 66–72.

McGuire, D. K., Levine, B. D., Williamson, J. W., Snell, P. G., Blomqvist, C. G., Saltin, B., and Mitchell, J. H. "A 30-Year Follow-Up of the Dallas Bedrest and Training Study: I. Effect of Age on Cardiovascular Response to Exercise." *Circulation* 104 (2001): 1350–57.

Tsuji, I., Tamagawa, A., Nagatomi, R., Irie, N., Ohkubo, T., Saito, M., Fujita, K., Ogawa, K., Sauvaget, C., Anzai, Y., Hozawa, A., Watanabe, Y., Sato, A., Ohmori, H., and Hisamichi, S. "Randomized Controlled Trial of Exercise

Training for Older People (Sendai Silver Center Trial; SSCT): Study Design and Primary Outcome." *Journal of Epidemiology* 10 (2000): 55–64.

Exercise and Ankylosing Spondylitis (AS)

Uhrin, Z., Kuzis, S., and Ward, M. M. "Exercise and Changes in Health Status in Patients with Ankylosing Spondylitis." *Archives of Internal Medicine* 160 (2000): 2969–75.

Exercise and Arrhythmias

Jensen-Urstad, K., Bouvier, F., Saltin, B., and Jensen-Urstad, M. "High Prevalence of Arrhythmias in Elderly Male Athletes with a Lifelong History of Regular Strenuous Exercise." *Heart* 79 (1998): 161–64.

Exercise and Behavior

Bock, B. C., Marcus, B. H., Pinto, B. M., and Forsyth, L. H. "Maintenance of Physical Activity Following an Individualized Motivationally Tailored Intervention." *Annals of Behavioral Medicine* 23 (2001): 79–87.

McAuley, E., Bane, S. M., and Mihalko, S. L. "Exercise in Middle-Aged Adults: Self-Efficacy and Self-Presentational Outcomes." *Preventive Medicine* 24 (1995): 319–28.

Oman, R. F., and King, A. C. "The Effect of Life Events and Exercise Program Format on the Adoption and Maintenance of Exercise Behavior." *Health Psychology* 19 (2000): 605–12.

Sherwood, N. E., and Jeffery, R. W. "The Behavioral Determinants of Exercise: Implications for Physical Activity Interventions." *Annual Reviews of Nutrition* (2000): 21–44.

Exercise and Blood Pressure

Dengel, D. R., Hagberg, J. M., Pratley, R. E., Rogus, E. M., and Goldberg, A. P. "Improvements in Blood Pressure, Glucose Metabolism, and Lipoprotein Lipids after Aerobic Exercise Plus Weight Loss in Obese, Hypertensive Middle-Aged Men." *Metabolism* 47 (1998): 1075–82.

Hayashi, T., Tsumura, K., Suematsu, C., Okada, K., Fujii, S., and Endo, G. "Walking to Work and the Risk for Hypertension in Men: The Osaka Health Survey." *Annals of Internal Medicine* 131 (1999): 21–26.

Young, D. R., Appel, L. J., Jee, S., and Miller, E. "The Effects of Aerobic Exercise and T'ai Chi on Blood Pressure in Older People: Results of a Randomized Trial." *Journal of the American Geriatrics Society* 47 (1999): 277–84.

Exercise and Cancer

Albanes, D., Blair, A., and Taylor, P. R. "Physical Activity and Risk of Cancer in the NHANES I Population." *American Journal of Public Health* 79 (1989): 744–50.

Giovannucci, E., Leitzmann, M., Spiegelman, D., Rimm, E. B., Colditz, G. A., Stampfer, M. J., and Willett, W. C. "A Prospective Study of Physical Activity and Prostate Cancer in Male Health Professionals." *Cancer Research* 58 (1998): 5117–22.

Liu, S., Lee, I. M., Linson, P., Ajani, U., Buring, J. E., and Hennekens, C. H. "A Prospective Study of Physical Activity and Risk of Prostate Cancer in U.S. Physicians." *International Journal of Epidemiology* 29 (2000): 29–35.

Lee, I. M., Manson, J. E., Ajani, U., Paffenbarger, R. S., Hennekens, C. H., and Buring, J. E. "Physical Activity and Risk of Colon Cancer: The Physicians' Health Study (United States)." *Cancer Causes and Control* 8 (1997): 568–74.

Michaud, D. S., Giovannucci, E., Willett, W. C., Colditz, G. A., Stampfer, M. J., and Fuchs, C. S. "Physical Activity, Obesity, Height, and the Risk of Pancreatic Cancer." *JAMA* 286 (2001): 921–29.

Platz, E., Kawachi, I., Rimm, E. B., Colditz, G. A., Stampfer, M. J., Willett, W. C., Giovannucci, E. "Physical Activity and Benign Prostatic Hyperplasia." *Archives of Internal Medicine* 158 (1998): 2349–56.

Thune, I., and Furberg, A. S. "Physical Activity and Cancer Risk: Dose-Response and Cancer, All Sites and Site-Specific." *Medicine and Science in Sports and Exercise* 33 (2001): S530–50.

Exercise and Cardiovascular Disease

Ades, P. A., Waldmann, M. L., Meyer, W. L., Brown, K. A., Poehlman, E. T., Pendlebury, W. W., Leslie, K. O., Gray, P. R., Lew, R. R., and LeWinter, M. M. "Skeletal Muscle and Cardiovascular Adaptations to Exercise Conditioning in Older Coronary Patients." *Circulation* 94 (1996): 323–30.

Bijnen, F. C., Caspersen, C. J., Feskens, E. J., Saris, W. H., Mosterd, W. L., and Kromhout, D. "Physical Activity and 10-Year Mortality from Cardiovascular Diseases and All Causes: The Zutphen Elderly Study." *Archives of Internal Medicine* 158 (1998): 1499–505.

Dunn, A. L., Marcus, B. H., Kampert, J. B., Garcia, M. E., Kohl, H. W., and Blair, S. N. "Comparison of Lifestyle and Structured Interventions to Increase Physical Activity and Cardiorespiratory Fitness: A Randomized Trial." *JAMA* 281 (1999): 327–34.

Gartside, P. S., Wang, P., and Glueck, C. J. "Prospective Assessment of Coronary Heart Disease Risk Factors: The NHANES I Epidemiologic Follow-Up Study (NHEFS) 16-Year Follow-Up. *Journal of the American College of Nutrition* 17 (1998): 263–69.

Hakim, A. A., Curb, D., Petrovitch, H., Rodriguez, B. L., Yano, K., Ross, G. W., White, L. R., and Abbott, R. D. "Effects of Walking on Coronary Heart Disease in Elderly Men: The Honolulu Heart Program." *Circulation* 100 (1999): 9–13.

Hu, F., Stampfer, M. J., Colditz, G. A., Ascherio, A., Rexrode, K. M., Willett, W. C., and Manson, J. E. "Physical Activity and Risk of Stroke in Women." *JAMA* 283 (2000): 2961–67.

LaMonte, M. J., Eisenman, P. A., Adams, T. D., Shultz, B. B., Ainsworth, B. E., and Yanowitz, F. G. "Cardiorespiratory Fitness and Coronary Heart Disease Risk Factors: The LDS Hospital Fitness Institute Cohort." *Circulation* 102 (2000): 1623–28.

Sesso, H. D., Paffenbarger, R. S., and Lee, I.-M. "Physical Activity and Coronary Heart Disease in Men: The Harvard Alumni Health Study." *Circulation* 102 (2000): 975–80.

Lee, I.-M., Sesso, H. D., and Paffenbarger, R. S. "Physical Activity and Coronary Heart Disease in Men: Does the Duration of Exercise Episodes Predict Risk?" *Circulation* 102 (2000): 981–86.

Manson, J. E., Hu, F. B., Rich-Edwards, J. W., Colditz, G. A, Stampfer, M. J., Willett, W. C., Speizer, F. E., and Hennekens, C. H. "A Prospective Study of Walking as Compared with Vigorous Exercise in the Prevention of Coronary Heart Disease in Women." *New England Journal of Medicine* 341 (1999): 650–58.

Shepard, R. J., and Balady, G. J. "Exercise as Cardiovascular Therapy." *Circulation* 99 (1999): 963–72.

Stofan, J. R., DiPietro, L., Davis, D., Kohl, H. W., Blair, S. N. "Physical Activity Patterns Associated with Cardiorespiratory Fitness and Reduced Mortality: The Aerobics Center Longitudinal Study." *American Journal of Public Health* 88 (1998): 1807–13.

Exercise and Cholesterol

Stefanick, M. L., Mackey, S., Sheehan, M., Ellsworth, N., Haskell, W. L., and Wood, P. D. "Effects of Diet and Exercise in Men and Postmenopausal Women with Low Levels of HDL Cholesterol and High Levels of LDL Cholesterol." *New England Journal of Medicine* 339 (1998): 12–20.

Exercise and Chronic Obstructive Pulmonary Disease

Finnerty, J. P., Keeping, I., Bullough, I., and Jones, J. "The Effectiveness of Outpatient Pulmonary Rehabilitation in Chronic Lung Disease." *Chest* 119 (2001): 1705–10.

Exercise and Cognitive Decline

Albert, M. S., Jones, K., Savage, C. R., Berkman, L., Seeman, T., Blazer, D., and Rowe, J. W. "Predictors of Cognitive Change in Older Persons: MacArthur Studies of Successful Aging." *Psychology and Aging* 10 (1995): 578–89.

Laurin, D., Verreault, R., Lindsay, J., MacPherson, K., and Rockwood, K. "Physical Activity and Risk of Cognitive Impairment and Dementia in Elderly Persons." *Archives of Neurology* 58 (2001): 498–504.

Yaffe, K., Barnes, D., Nevitt, M., Lui, L.-Y., and Covinsky, K. "A Prospective Study of Physical Activity and Cognitive Decline in Elderly Women." *Archives of Internal Medicine* 161 (2001): 1703–8.

Exercise and Diabetes

Hu, F. B., Leitzmann, M. F., Stampfer, M. J., Colditz, G. A., Willett, W. C., and Rimm, E. B. "Physical Activity and Television Watching in Relation to Risk for Type 2 Diabetes Mellitus in Men." *Archives of Internal Medicine* 161 (2001): 1542–48.

Hu, F. B., Sigal, R. J., Rich-Edwards, J. W., Colditz, G. A., Solomon, C. G., Willett, W. C., Speizer, F. E., and Manson, J. E. "Walking Compared with Vigorous Physical Activity and Risk of Type 2 Diabetes in Women: A Prospective Study." *JAMA* 282 (1999): 1433–39.

Manson, J. E., Nathan, D. M., Krolewski, A. S., Stampfer, M. J., Willett, W. C., and Hennekens, C. H. "A Prospective Study of Exercise and Incidence of Diabetes among U.S. Male Physicians." *JAMA* 268 (1992): 63–67.

Takemura, Y., Kikuchi, S., Inaba, Y., Yasuda, H., and Nakagawa, K. "The Protective Effect of Good Physical Fitness When Young on the Risk of Impaired Glucose Tolerance When Old." *Preventive Medicine* (1999): 14–19.

Tuomilehto, J., Lindström, J., Eriksson, J. G., Valle, T. T., Hämäläinen, H., Ilanne-Parikka, P., Keinänen-Kiukaanniemi, S., Laakso, M., Louheranta, A., Rastas, M., Salminen, V., and Uusitupa, M., for the Finnish Diabetes Prevention Study Group. "Prevention of Type 2 Diabetes Mellitus by Changes in Lifestyle among Subjects with Impaired Glucose Tolerance." *New England Journal of Medicine* 344 (2001): 1343–50.

Exercise and Gallstones

Leitzman, M. F., Rimm, E. B., Willett, W. C., Spiegelman, D., Grodstein, F., Stampfer, M. J., Colditz, G. A., and Giovannucci, E. "Recreational Physical Activity and the Risk of Cholecystectomy in Women." *New England Journal of Medicine* 341 (1999): 777–84.

Exercise and Longevity

Bijen, F. C., Feskens, E. J., Caspersen, C. J., Nagelkerke, N., Mosterd, W. L., and Kromhout, D. "Baseline and Previous Physical Activity in Relation to Mortality in Elderly Men: The Zutphen Elderly Study." *American Journal of Epidemiology* 150 (1999): 1289–96.

Erikssen, G., Liestol, K., Bjornholt, J., Thaulow, E., Sandvik, L., and Erikssen, J. "Changes in Physical Fitness and Changes in Mortality." *Lancet* 352 (1998): 759–62.

Hakim, A. A., Petrovitch, H., Burchfiel, C. M., Ross, G. W., Rodriguez, B. L., White, L. R., Yano, K., Curb, J. D., and Abbott, R. D. "Effects of Walking on Mortality among Nonsmoking Retired Men." *New England Journal of Medicine* 338 (1998): 94–99.

Kaplan, G. A., Seeman, T. E., Cohen, R. D., Knudsen, L. P., and Guralnik, J. "Mortality Among the Elderly in the Alameda County Study: Behavioral and

Demographic Risk Factors." *American Journal of Public Health* 77 (1987): 307–212.

Lee, I.-M., and Paffenbarger, R. S. "Associations between Light, Moderate and Vigorous Intensity Activity with Longevity: The Harvard Alumni Health Study." *American Journal of Epidemiology* 151 (2000): 293–99.

Lee, I.-M., Hsieh, C. C., and Paffenbarger, R. S. "Exercise Intensity and Longevity in Men: The Harvard Alumni Health Study." *JAMA* 273 (1995): 1179–84.

Paffenbarger, R. S., Hyde, R. T., Wing, A. L., Lee, I.-M., Jung, D. L., and Kampert, J. B. "The Association of Changes in Physical-Activity Level and Other Lifestyle Characteristics with Mortality Among Men." *New England Journal of Medicine* 328 (1993): 538–45.

Paffenbarger, R. S., Hyde, R. T., Wing. A. L., and Hsieh, C. C. "Physical Activity, All-Cause Mortality, and Longevity of College Alumni." *New England Journal of Medicine* 314 (1986): 605–13.

Rockhill, B., Willett, W. C., Manson, J. E., Leitzmann, M. F., Stampfer, M. J., Hunter, D. J., and Colditz, G. A. "Physical Activity and Mortality: A Prospective Study among Women." *American Journal of Public Health* 91 (2001): 578–83.

Sandvik, L., Erikssen, J., Thaulow, E., Erikssen, G., Mundal, R., and Rodahl, K. "Physical Fitness as a Predictor of Mortality among Healthy, Middle-Aged Norwegian Men." *New England Journal of Medicine* 328 (1993): 533–37.

Weight Training and Heart Disease

Maiorana, A., O'Driscoll, G., Dembo, L., Cheetham, C., Goodman, C., Taylor, R., and Green, D. "Effect of Aerobic and Resistance Exercise Training on Vascular Function in Heart Failure." *American Journal of Physiology—Heart & Circulatory Physiology* 279 (2000): H1999–2005.

McCartney, N. "Role of Resistance Training in Heart Disease." *Medicine and Science in Sports and Exercise* 30 (1998): S396–402.

Pu, C. T., Johnson, M. T., Forman, D. E., Hausdorff, J. M., Roubenoff, R., Foldvari, M., Fielding, R. A., and Fiatarone Singh, M. A. "Randomized Trial of Progressive Resistance Training to Counteract the Myopathy of Chronic Heart Failure." *Journal of Applied Physiology* 90 (2001): 2341–50.

Weight Training and Osteoporosis

Hunter, G. R., Wetzstein, C. J., McLafferty, C. L., Zuckerman, P. A., Landers, K. A., and Bamman, M. M. "High-Resistance Versus Variable-Resistance Training in Older Adults." *Medicine and Science in Sports and Exercise* 33 (2001): 1759–64.

Kerr, D., Ackland, T., Maslen, B., Morton, A., and Prince, R. "Resistance Training over 2 Years Increases Bone Mass in Calcium-Replete Post-menopausal Women." *Journal of Bone and Mineral Research* 16 (2001): 175–81.

Layne, J., and Nelson, M. E. "The Effects of Progressive Resistance Training on Bone Density: A Review." *Medicine and Science in Sports and Exercise* 31 (1999): 25–30.

Weight Training and Other Diseases

Castaneda, C., Gordon, P. L., Uhlin, K. L., Levey, A. S., Kehayias, J. J., Dwyer, J. T., Fielding, R. A., Roubenoff, R., and Singh, M. F. "Resistance Training to Counteract the Catabolism of a Low-Protein Diet in Patients with Chronic Renal Insufficiency: A Randomized, Controlled Trial." *Annals of Internal Medicine* 135 (2001): 965–76.

Copley, J. B. "Resistance Training Enhances the Value of Protein Restriction in the Treatment of Chronic Kidney Disease." *Annals of Internal Medicine* 135 (2001): 999–1001.

Häkkinen, A., Sokka, T., Kotaniemi, A., and Hannonen, P. "A Randomized Two-Year Study of the Effects of Dynamic Strength Training on Muscle Strength, Disease Activity, Functional Capacity, and Bone Mineral Density in Early Rheumatoid Arthritis." *Arthritis and Rheumatism* 44 (2001): 515–22.

Scandalis, T. A., Bosak, A., Berliner, J. C., Helman, L. L., and Wells, M. R. "Resistance Training and Gait Function in Patients with Parkinson's Disease." *American Journal of Physical Medicine and Rehabilitation* 80 (2001): 38–43.

Weight Training in Older Persons

Fiatarone, M. A., O'Neill, E. F., Doyle Ryan, N., Clements, K. M., Solares, G. R., Nelson, M. E., Roberts, S. B., Kehayias, J. J., Lipsitz, L. A., and Evans, W. J. "Exercise Training and Nutritional Supplementation for Physical Frailty in Very Elderly People." *New England Journal of Medicine* 330 (1994): 1769–75.

Fiatarone, M. A., Marks, E. C., Ryan, N. D., Meredith, C. N., Lipsitz, L. A., and Evans, W. J. "High-Intensity Strength Training in Nonagenarians: Effects on Skeletal Muscle." *JAMA* (1990): 3029–34.

Hurley, B. F., and Roth, S. M. "Strength Training in the Elderly: Effects on Risk Factors for Age-Related Diseases." *Sports Medicine* 30 (2000): 249–68.

Kelley, G. A., and Sharpe Kelley, K. "Progressive Resistance Exercise and Resting Blood Pressure: A Meta-Analysis of Randomized Controlled Trials." *Hypertension* 35 (2000): 838–43.

Melton, L. J., Khosla, S., Crowson, C. S., O'Connor, M. K., O'Fallon, W. M., and Riggs, B. L. "Epidemiology of Sarcopenia." *Journal of the American Geriatrics Society* 48 (2000): 625–30.

Pollock, M. L., and Evans, W. J. "Resistance Training for Health and Disease: Introduction." *Medicine and Science in Sports and Exercise* 31 (1999): 10–11.

Sclicht, J. Camaione, D. N., and Owen, S. V. "Effect of Intense Strength Training on Standing Balance, Walking Speed, and Sit-to-Stand Performance in Older Adults." *Journals of Gerontology: Biological Sciences & Medical Sciences* 56A (2001): M281–86.

Winett, R. A., and Carpinelli, R. N. "Potential Health-Related Benefits of Resistance Training." *Preventive Medicine* 33 (2001): 503–13.

Chapter 4

General

Allison, D. B., Fontaine, K. R., Manson, J. E., Stevens, J., and Van Itallie, T. B. "Annual Deaths Attributable to Obesity in the United States." *JAMA* 282 (1999): 1530–538.

Insel, P., Turner, R. E., and Ross, D. *Nutrition.* 2002 update. (2002). Boston: Jones and Barlett Publishers.

Katch, F. I., and McArdle, W. D. *Introduction to Nutrition, Exercise, and Health.* 4th ed. (1993). Baltimore: Williams & Wilkins.

Leibel, R. L., Rosenbaum, M., and Hirsch, J. "Changes in Energy Expenditure Resulting from Altered Body Weight." *New England Journal of Medicine* 332 (1995): 621–28.

National Heart, Lung, and Blood Institute. "Clinical Guidelines on the Identi-fication, Evaluation, and Treatment of Overweight and Obesity in Adults: Executive Summary." *National Institutes of Health* (May 2001): NIH Publica-tion Number 01-3670.

National Heart, Lung, and Blood Institute. "The Practical Guide: Identifi-cation, Evaluation, and Treatment of Overweight and Obesity in Adults." *National Institutes of Health* (October 2000): NIH Publication Number 00-4084.

National Task Force on the Prevention and Treatment of Obesity. "Weight Cy-cling." *JAMA* 272 (1994): 1196–202.

St. Jeor, S. T., Howard, B. V., Prewitt, E., Bovee, V., Bazzarre, T., and Eckel, R. H., for the AHA Nutrition Committee. "Dietary Protein and Weight Reduction: A Statement for Healthcare Professionals from the Nutrition Committee of the Council on Nutrition, Physical Activity, and Metabolism of the Amer-ican Heart Association." *Circulation* 104 (2001): 1869–874.

U.S. Department of Health and Human Services. "The Surgeon General's Call to Action to Prevent and Decrease Overweight and Obesity." Rockville, MD: U.S. Department of Health and Human Services, Public Health Service, Of-fice of the Surgeon General (2001).

Caloric Restriction

Masoro, E. J. "Caloric Restriction and Aging: An Update." *Experimental Geron-tology* 35 (2000): 299–305.

Sohal, R. S., and Weindruch, R. "Oxidative Stress, Caloric Restriction, and Aging." *Science* 273 (1996): 59–63.

Walford, R. L. *The 120-Year Diet: How to Double Your Vital Years.* (1986) New York: Simon and Schuster.

Weindruch, R. "Effect of Caloric Restriction on Age-Associated Cancers." *Ex-perimental Gerontology* 27 (1992): 575–81.

Weight and Diseases

Field, A. E., Coakley, E. H., Must, A., Spadano, J. L., Laird, N., Dietz, W. H., Rimm, E., and Colditz, G. A. "Impact of Overweight on the Risk of Devel-oping Common Chronic Diseases during a 10-Year Period." *Archives of In-ternal Medicine* 161 (2001): 1581–86.

Ford, E. S., Giles, W. H., and Dietz, W. H. "Prevalence of the Metabolic Syndrome Among U.S. Adults: Findings from the Third National Health and Nutrition Examination Survey." *JAMA* 287 (2002): 356–59.

Weight and Hip Fractures

Ensrud, K. E., Cauley, J., Lipschutz, R., and Cummings, S. R. "Weight Change and Fractures in Older Women." *Archives of Internal Medicine* 157 (1997): 857–63.

Ensrud, K. E., Lipschutz, R., Cauley, J., Seely, D., Nevitt, M. C., Orwoll, E. S., Genant, H. K., and Cummings, S. R. "Body Size and Hip Fracture Risk in Older Women: A Prospective Study. Study of Osteoporotic Fractures Research Group." *American Journal of Medicine* 103 (1997): 274–80.

Farahmand, B. Y., Michaëlsson, K., Baron, J. A., Persson, P.-G., and Ljunghall, S., for the Swedish Hip Fracture Study Group. "Body Size and Hip Fractures Risk." *Epidemiology* 11 (2000): 214–19.

Meyer, H. E., Tverdal, A., and Selmer, R. "Weight Variability, Weight Change and the Incidence of Hip Fracture: A Prospective Study of 39,000 Middle-Aged Norwegians." *Osteoporosis International* 8 (1998): 373–78.

Weight and Longevity

Calle, E. E., Thun, M. J., Petrelli, J. M., Rodriguez, C., and Heath, C. W. "Body-Mass Index and Mortality in a Prospective Cohort of U.S. Adults." *New England Journal of Medicine* 341 (1999): 1097–105.

Folsom, A. R., Kaye, S. A., Sellers, T. A., Hong, C.-P., Cerhan, J. R., Potter, J. D., and Prineas, R. J. "Body Fat Distribution and 5-Year Risk of Death in Older Women." *JAMA* 269 (1993): 483–87.

Grabowski, D. C., and Ellis, J. E. "High Body Mass Index Does Not Predict Mortality in Older People: Analysis of the Longitudinal Study of Aging." *Journal of the American Geriatrics Society* 49 (2001): 968–79.

Hanson, R. L., McCance, D. R., Jacobsson, L. T., Narayan, K. M., Nelson, R. G., Pettitt, D. J., Bennett, P. H., and Knowler, W. C. "The U-Shaped Association between Body Mass Index and Mortality: Relationship with Weight Gain in a Native American Population." *Journal of Clinical Epidemiology* 48 (1995): 903–16.

Kuczmarski, R. J., Carroll, M. D., Flegal, K. M., and Troiano, R. P. "Varying Body Mass Index Cutoff Points to Describe Overweight Prevalence Among U.S. Adults: NHANES III (1988 to 1994)." *Obesity Research* 5 (1997): 542–48.

Lee, I.-M., Manson, J. E., Hennekens, C. H., and Paffenbarger, R. S. "Body Weight and Mortality: A 27-Year Follow-Up of Middle-Aged Men." *JAMA* 270 (1993): 2823–28.

Mikkelsen, K. L., Heitmann, B. L., Keiding, N., and Sorensen, T. I. "Independent Effects of Stable and Changing Body Weight on Total Mortality." *Epidemiology* (1999): 671–78.

Reynolds, M. W., Fredman, L., Langenberg, P., and Magaziner, J. "Weight, Weight Change, and Mortality in a Random Sample of Older Community-Dwelling Women." *Journal of the American Geriatrics Society* 47 (1999): 1409–14.

Weight-Loss Drugs

Abenhaim, L., Moride, Y., Brenot, F., Rich, S., Benichou, J., Kurz, X., Higenbottam, T., Oakley, C., Wouters, E., Aubier, M., Simonneau, G., and Bégaud, B., for the International Primary Pulmonary Hypertension Study Group. "Appetite-Suppressant Drugs and the Risk of Primary Pulmonary Hypertension." *New England Journal of Medicine* 335 (1996): 609–16.

Blanck, H. M., Khan, L. K., and Serdula, M. K. "Use of Nonprescription Weight-Loss Products: Results from a Multistate Survey." *JAMA* 286 (2001): 930–5.

Fellow, E. "Ephedra/Ephedrine: Cardiovascular and CNS Effects." *Canadian Medical Association Journal* 166 (2002): 633.

Haller, C. A., and Benowitz, N. L. "Adverse Cardiovascular and Central Nervous System Events Associated with Dietary Supplements Containing Ephedra Alkaloids." *New England Journal of Medicine* 343 (2000): 1833–38.

Rich, S., Rubin, L., Walker, A. M., Schneeweiss, S., and Abenhaim, L. "Anorexigens and Pulmonary Hypertension in the United States—Results from the Surveillance of North American Pulmonary Hypertension." *Chest* 117 (2000): 870–4.

Weight-Loss Maintenance

Anderson, J. W., Konz, E. C., Frederich, R. C., and Wood, C. L. "Long-Term Weight-Loss Maintenance: A Meta-Analysis of U.S. Studies." *American Journal of Clinical Nutrition* 74 (2001): 579–84.

Wing, R. R., and Hill, J. O. "Successful Weight-Loss Maintenance." *Annual Reviews of Nutrition* 21 (2001): 323–41.

Chapter 5

Ancoli-Israel, S. *All I Want Is a Good Night's Sleep.* (1996). St. Louis: Mosby-Year Book, Inc.

Dement, W. C., and Vaughn, C. *The Promise of Sleep.* (1999) New York: Dell Publishing.

Folks, D. G., and Fuller, W. C. "Anxiety Disorders and Insomnia in Geriatric Patients." *Psychiatric Clinics of North America* 20 (1997): 137–64.

National Highway Traffic Safety Administration and National Center on Sleep Disorders Research. "Drowsy Driving and Automobile Crashes: Report and Recommendations." (April 1998). DOT Publication No. 808 707. Washington, DC, and Bethesda, MD.

National Institute of Mental Health. "The Numbers Count: Mental Disorders in America." (January 2001). NIMH Publication No. 01-4584. Bethesda, MD.

National Institute of Neurological Disorders and Stroke. "Brain Basics: Understanding Sleep." (July 2001). www.ninds.nih.gov/health–and–medical/pubs/understanding–sleep–brain–basic–.htm#Sleep Disorders

National Sleep Foundation. "2000 Omnibus Sleep in America Poll (OSAP)." (2000). www.sleepfoundation.org/publications/2000poll.html

National Sleep Foundation. "Events of 9-11 Took Their Toll on Americans' Sleep . . ." (November 19, 2001). www.sleepfoundation.org/whatsnew/crisis–poll.html

National Sleep Foundation. "Facts about PLMS." www.sleepfoundation.org/publications/fact–plms.html

Van Cauter, E., Leproult, R., and Plat, L. "Age-Related Changes in Slow Wave Sleep and REM Sleep and Relationship with Growth Hormone and Cortisol Levels in Healthy Men." *JAMA* 284 (2000): 861–68.

Yang, C. M., Spielman, A. J., D'Ambrosio, P., Serizawa, S., Nunes, J., and Birnbaum, J. "A Single Dose of Melatonin Prevents the Phase Delay Associated with a Delayed Weekend Sleep Pattern." *Sleep* 24 (2001): 272–81.

Chapter 6

General

Burns, G. *How to Live to Be 100—or More: The Ultimate Diet, Sex, and Exercise Book.* (1989). New York: Plume.

Redelmeier, D. Singh, S. "Survival in Academy Award-Winning Actors and Actresses." *Annals of Internal Medicine* 134 (2001): 1001–3.

Anger

Kawachi, I., Sparrow, D., Spiro, A., Vokonas, P., and Weiss, S. T. "A Prospective Study of Anger and Coronary Heart Disease. The Normative Aging Study." *Circulation* 94 (1996): 2090–5.

Depression (General)

Hays, J. C., Landerman, L. R., George, L. K., Flint, E. P., Koenig, H. G., Land, K. C., and Blazer, D. G. "Social Correlates of the Dimensions of Depression in the Elderly." *Journal of Gerontology: Psychological Sciences and Social Sciences* 53 (1998): P31–39.

Huang, B. Y., Cornoni-Huntley, J., Hays, J. C., Huntley, R. R., Galanos, A. N., and Blazer, D. G. "Impact of Depressive Symptoms on Hospitalization Risk in Community-Dwelling Older Persons." *Journal of the American Geriatrics Society* 48 (2000): 1279–84.

Steffens, D. C., Hays, J. C., and Krishnan, K. R. R. "Disability in Geriatric Depression." *American Journal of Geriatric Psychiatry* 7 (1999): 34–40.

Vogt, T., Pope, C., Mullooly, J., and Hollis, J. "Mental Health Status as a Predictor of Morbidity and Mortality: A 15-Year Follow-Up of Members of a Health Maintenance Organization." *American Journal of Public Health* 84 (1994): 227–31.

Wulsin, L. R. "Does Depression Kill?" *Archives of Internal Medicine* 160 (2000): 1731–32.

Depression and Bones

Schweiger, U., Deuschle, M., Korner, A., Lammers, C. H., Schmider, J., Gotthardt, U., Holsboer, F., and Heuser, I. "Low Lumbar Bone Mineral Density in Patients with Major Depression." *American Journal of Psychiatry* 151 (1994): 1691–93.

Depression and Heart Disease

Barefoot, J. C., Helms, M. J., Mark, D. B., Blumenthal, J. A., Califf, R. M., Haney, T. L., O'Connor, C. M., Siegler, I. C., and Williams, R. B. "Depression and Long-Term Mortality Risk in Patients with Coronary Artery Disease." *American Journal of Cardiology* 78 (1996): 613–17.

Cameron, O. "Depression Increases Post-MI Mortality: How?" *Psychosomatic Medicine* 58 (1996): 111–12.

Carney, R. M., Blumenthal, J. A., Stein, P. K., Watkins, L., Catellier, D., Berkman, L. F., Czajkowski, S. M., O'Connor, C., Stone, P. H., and Freedland, K. E. "Depression, Heart Rate Variability, and Acute Myocardial Infarction." *Circulation* 104 (2001): 2024–28.

Frasure-Smith, N., Bourassa, M. G. "Social Support, Depression, and Mortality during the First Year after Myocardial Infarction." *Circulation* 101 (2000): 1919–24.

Fransure-Smith, N., Lespérance, F., and Talajic, M., "Depression and 18-Month Prognosis after Myocardial Infarction." *Circulation* 91 (1995): 999–1005.

Krittayaphong, R., Cascio, W. E., Light, K. C., Sheffield, D., Golden, R. N., Finkel, J. B., Glekas, G., Koch, G. G., and Sheps, D. S. "Heart Rate Variability in Patients with Coronary Artery Disease: Differences in Patients with Higher and Lower Depression Scores." *Psychosomatic Medicine* 59 (1997): 231–35.

Depression and Stroke

Colantonio, A., Kasi, S. V., and Ostfeld, A. M. "Depressive Symptoms and Other Psychosocial Factors as Predictors of Stroke in the Elderly." *American Journal of Epidemiology* 136 (1992): 884–94.

Everson, S. A., Roberts, R. E., Goldberg, D. E., and Kaplan, G. A. "Depressive Symptoms and Increased Risk of Stroke Mortality over a 29-Year Period." *Archives of Internal Medicine* 158 (1998): 1133–8.

Education

Crimmins, E. M., and Saito, Y. "Trends in Healthy Life Expectancy in the United States, 1970–1990: Gender, Racial, and Educational Differences." *Social Science and Medicine* 52 (2001): 1629–41.

Lauderdale, D. S. "Education and Survival: Birth Cohort, Period, and Age Effects." *Demography* 38 (2001): 551–61.

Ross, C. E., and Wu, C.-L. "Education, Age, and the Cumulative Advantage to Health." *Journal of Health and Social Behavior* 37 (1996): 104–20.

Ross, C. E., and Wu, C.-L. "The Links Between Education and Health." *American Sociological Review* 60 (1995): 719–45.

Meditation

Cunningham, C., Brown, S., and Kaski, J. C. "Effects of Transcendental Meditation on Symptoms and Electrocardiographic Changes in Patients with Cardiac Syndrome X." *American Journal of Cardiology* 85 (2000): 653–55.

Snaith, P. "Meditation and Psychotherapy." *British Journal of Psychiatry* 173 (1998): 193–95.

Zamarra, J. W., Schneider, R. H., Besseghini, I., Robinson, D. K., Salerno, J. W. "Usefulness of the Transcendental Meditation Program in the Treatment of Patients with Coronary Artery Disease." *American Journal of Cardiology* 77 (1996): 867–70.

Optimism

Mulkana, S. S., and Hailey, B. J. "The Role of Optimism in Health-Enhancing Behavior." *American Journal of Health Behavior* 25 (2001): 388–95.

Achat, H., Kawachi, I., Spiro, A., DeMolles, D. A., and Sparrow, D. "Optimism and Depression as Predictors of Physical and Mental Health Functioning: The Normative Aging Study." *Annals of Behavioral Medicine* 22 (2000): 127–30.

Religion & Spirituality

Ellison, C. G. "Race, Religious Involvement and Depressive Symptomatology in a Southeastern U. S. Community." *Social Science and Medicine* 40 (1995): 1561–72.

Helm, H. M., Hays, J. C., Flint, E. P., Koenig, H. G., and Blazer, D. G. "Does Private Religious Activity Prolong Survival? A Six-Year Follow-Up Study of 3,851 Older Adults." *Journal of Gerontology: Biological Sciences and Medical Sciences* 55 (2000): M400–5.

Koenig, H. G., Hays, J. C., Larson, D. B., George, L. K., Cohen, H. J., McCullough, M. E., Meador, K. G., and Blazer, D. G. "Does Religious Attendance Prolong Survival? A Six-Year Follow-Up Study of 3,968 Older Adults." *Journal of Gerontology: Biological Sciences and Medical Sciences* 54 (1999): M670–6.

Koenig, H. G., George, L. K., Hays, J. C., Larson, D. B., Cohen, H. J., and Blazer, D. G. "The Relationship Between Religious Activities and Blood Pressure in Older Adults." *International Journal of Psychiatry in Medicine* 28 (1998): 189–213.

Koenig, H. G., Cohen, H. J., George, L. K., Hays, J. C., Larson, D. B., and Blazer, D. G. "Attendance at Religious Services, Interleukin-6, and Other Biological Parameters of Immune Function in Older Adults." *International Journal of Psychiatry in Medicine* 27 (1997): 233–50.

Koenig, H. G., Hays, J. C., George, L. K., Blazer, D. G., Larson, D. B., and Landerman, L. R. "Modeling the Cross-Sectional Relationships Between Religion, Physical Health, Social Support, and Depressive Symptoms." *American Journal of Geriatric Psychiatry* 5 (1997): 131–44.

Koenig, H. G., Cohen, H. J., Blazer, D. G., Kudler, H. S., Krishnan, K. R., and Sibert, T. E. "Religious Coping and Cognitive Symptoms of Depression in Elderly Medical Patients." *Psychosomatics* 36 (1995): 369–75.

Strawbridge, W. J., Shema, S. J., Cohen, R. D., and Kaplan, G. A. "Religious Attendance Increases Survival by Improving and Maintaining Good Health Behaviors, Mental Health, and Social Relationships." *Annals of Behavioral Medicine* 23 (2001): 68–74.

Sex (General)

Dunn, K. M., Croft, P. R., and Hackett, G. I. "Association of Sexual Problems with Social, Psychological, and Physical Problems in Men and Women: A Cross Sectional Population Study. *Journal of Epidemiology and Community Health* 53 (1999): 144–48.

Rosen, R. C., Lane, R. M., and Menza, J. "Effects of SSRIs on Sexual Function: A Critical Review." *Journal of Clinical Psychopharmacology* 19 (1999): 67–85.

Sex and Aging

Butler, R. N., and Lewis, M. I. "Sexuality and Aging." In: *Principles of Geriatric Medicine and Gerontology* (Hazzard, W. R., Blass, J. P., Ettinger, W. H., Halter, J. B., and Ouslander, J. G., eds. 4th ed. New York: McGraw-Hill. 1999.)

National Council on Aging. "Healthy Sexuality and Vital Aging." Washington, D.C.: author. 1998.

Weidner, W., Altwein, J., Hauck, E., Beutel, M, and Brähler, E. "Sexuality of the Elderly." *Urologia Internationalis* 66 (2001): 181–84.

Sex and Erectile Dysfunction

Araujo, A. B., Johannes, C. B., Feldman, H. A., Derby, C. A., and McKinlay, J. B. "Relation between Psychosocial Risk Factors and Incident Erectile Dysfunction: Prospective Results from the Massachusetts Male Aging Study." *American Journal of Epidemiology* 152 (2000): 533–41.

Araujo, A. B., Durante, R., Feldman, H. A., Goldstein, I., and McKinlay, J. B. "The Relationship between Depressive Symptoms and Male Erectile Dysfunction: Cross-Sectional Results from the Massachusetts Male Aging Study." *Psychosomatic Medicine* 60 (1998): 458–65.

Aytac, I. A., Araujo, A. B., Johannes, C. B., Kleinman, K. P., and McKinlay, J. B. "Socioeconomic Factors and Incidence of Erectile Dysfunction: Findings of the Longitudinal Massachusetts Male Aging Study." *Social Science and Medicine* 51 (2000): 771–78.

Cohan, P., and Korenman, S. G. "Erectile Dysfunction." *Journal of Clinical Endocrinology and Metabolism* 86 (2001): 2391–94.

Goldstein, I., Lue, T. F., Padma-Nathan, H., Rosen, R. C., Steers, W. D., and Wicker, P. A., for the Sildenafil Study Group. "Oral Sildenafil in the Treatment of Erectile Dysfunction." *New England Journal of Medicine* 338 (1998): 1397–404.

Gregoire, A. "Viagra: On Release." *British Medical Journal* 317 (1998): 759–60.

Johannes, C. B., Araujo, A. B., Feldman, H. A., Derby, C. A., Kleinman, K. P., and McKinlay, J. B. "Incidence of Erectile Dysfunction in Men 40 to 69 Years Old: Longitudinal Results from the Massachusetts Male Aging Study." *Journal of Urology* 163 (2000): 460–3.

Lue, T. F. "Erectile Dysfunction." *New England Journal of Medicine* 342 (2000): 1802–13.

Manecke, R. G., and Mulhall, J. P. "Medical Treatment of Erectile Dysfunction." *Annals of Medicine* 31 (1999): 388–98.

Nehra, A. "Treatment of Endocrinologic Male Sexual Dysfunction." *Mayo Clinic Proceedings* 75 Suppl (2000): S40–45.

Sex and Men

Bartlik, B., and Goldstein, M. Z. "Men's Sexual Health after Midlife." *Psychiatric Services* 52 (2001): 291–306.

Bortz, W. M., Wallace, D. H., and Wiley, D. "Sexual Function in 1,202 Aging Males: Differentiating Aspects." *Journals of Gerontology: Biological and Medical Sciences* 54 (1999): M237–41.

Kandeel, F. R., Koussa, V. K. T., and Swerdloff, R. S. "Male Sexual Function and Its Disorders: Physiology, Pathophysiology, Clinical Investigation, and Treatment." *Endocrine Reviews* 22 (2001): 342–88.

Sex and Women

Cawood, E. H. H., and Bancroft, J. "Steroid Hormones, the Menopause, Sexuality and Well-Being of Women." *Psychological Medicine* 26 (1996): 925–36.

Dennerstein, L., Dudley, E., and Burger, H. "Are Changes in Sexual Functioning during Midlife Due to Aging or Menopause?" *Fertility and Sterility* 76 (2001): 456–60.

Dennerstein, L., Dudley, E. C., Hopper, J. L., and Burger, H. "Sexuality, Hormones and the Menopausal Transition." *Maturitas* 26 (1997): 83–93.

Social Isolation and Ties

Fabrigoule, C., Letenneur, L., Dartigues, J. F., Zarrouk, M., Commenges, D., and Barberger-Gateau, P. "Social and Leisure Activities and Risk of Dementia: A Prospective Longitudinal Study." *Journal of the American Geriatrics Society* 43 (1995): 485–90.

Gliksman, M. D., Lazarus, R., Wilson, A., and Leeder, S. R. "Social Support, Marital Status and Living Arrangement Correlates of Cardiovascular Disease Risk Factors in the Elderly." *Social Science and Medicine* 40 (1995): 811–14.

Hays, J. C., Saunders, W. B., Flint, E. P., Kaplan, B. H., and Blazer, D. G. "Social Support and Depression as Risk Factors for Loss of Physical Function in Late Life." *Aging and Mental Health* 1 (1997): 209–20.

Litwin, H. "Social Network Type and Morale in Old Age." *Gerontologist* 41 (2001): 516–24.

Unger, J. B., McAvay, G., Bruce, M. L., Berkman, L., and Seeman, T. "Variation in the Impact of Social Network Characteristics on Physical Functioning in Elderly Persons: MacArthur Studies of Successful Aging." *Journal of Gerontology: Psychological and Social Sciences* 54 (1999): S245–51.

Chapter 7

Androstenedione

King, D. S., Sharp, R. L., Vukovich, M. D., Brown, G. A., Reifenrath, T. A., Uhl, N. L., and Parsons, K. A. "Effect of Oral Androstenedione on Serum Testosterone and Adaptations to Resistance Training in Young Men: A Randomized Controlled Trial." *JAMA* 281 (1999): 2020–28.

Rasmussen, B. B., Volpi, E., Gore, D. C., and Wolfe, R. R. "Androstenedione Does Not Stimulate Muscle Protein Anabolism in Young Healthy Men." *Journal of Clinical Endocrinology and Metabolism* 85 (2000): 55–59.

DHEA

Arlt, W., Callies, F., Koehler, I., van Vlijmen, J. C., Fassnacht, M., Strasburger, C. J., Seibel, M. J., Heubler, D., Ernst, M., Oettel, M., Reincke, M., Schulte, H. M., and Allolio, B. "Dehydroepiandrosterone Supplementation in Healthy Men with an Age-Related Decline of Dehydroepiandrosterone Secretion." *Journal of Clinical Endocrinology and Metabolism* 86 (2001): 4686–92.

Flynn, M. A., Weaver-Osterholtz, D. Sharpe-Timms, K. L., Allen, S., and Krause, G. "Dehydroepiandrosterone Replacement in Aging Humans." *Journal of Clinical Endocrinology and Metabolism* 84 (1999): 1527–33.

Trivedi, D. P., and Khaw, K. T. "Dehydroepiandrosterone Sulfate and Mortality in Elderly Men and Women." *Journal of Clinical Endocrinology and Metabolism* 86 (2001): 4171–77.

Estrogen

Al-Azzawi, F. "The Menopause and Its Treatment in Perspective." *Postgraduate Medical Journal* 77 (2001): 292–304.

Barrett-Connor, E. "Hormone Replacement Therapy." *British Medical Journal* 317 (1998): 457–61.

Chen, C-L., Weiss, N. S., Newcomb, P., Barlow, W., and White, E. "Hormone Replacement Therapy in Relation to Breast Cancer." *JAMA* 287 (2002): 734–41.

Collaborative Group on Hormonal Factors in Breast Cancer. "Breast Cancer and Hormone Replacement Therapy: Collaborative Reanalysis of Data from 51 Epidemiological Studies of 52,705 Women without Breast Cancer." *Lancet* 350 (1997): 1047–59.

Curran, M. P., and Wagstaff, A. J. "Estradiol and Norgestimate: A Review of Their Combined Use As Hormone Replacement Therapy in Post-menopausal Women." *Drugs and Aging* 18 (2001): 863–85.

Fletcher, S. W. and Colditz, G. A. "Failure of Estrogen Plus Progestin Therapy for Prevention." *JAMA* 288 (2002): 366–68.

Grady, D., Wenger, N. K., Herrington, D., Khan, S., Furberg, C., Hunninghake, D., Vittinghoff, E., Hulley, S., and the Heart and Estrogen/Progestin Replacement Study Research Group. "Postmenopausal Hormone Therapy Increases Risk for Venous Thromboembolic Disease. The Heart and Estrogen/Progestin Replacement Study." *Annals of Internal Medicine* 132 (2000): 689–96.

Grodstein, F., Manson, J. E., Colditz, G. A., Willett, W. C., Speizer, F. E., and Stampfer, M. J. "A Prospective, Observational Study of Postmenopausal Hormone Therapy and Primary Prevention of Cardiovascular Disease." *Annals of Internal Medicine* 133 (2000): 933–41.

Heckbert, S. R., Kaplan, R. C., Weiss, N. S., Psaty, B. M., Lin, D., Furberg, C. D., Starr, J. R., Anderson, G. D., and LaCroix, A. Z. "Risk of Recurrent Coronary Events in Relation to Use and Recent Initiation of Postmenopausal Hormone Therapy." *Archives of Internal Medicine* 161 (2001): 1709–13.

Herrington, D. M., Reboussin, D. M., Brosnihan, B., Sharp, P. C., Shumaker, S. A., Snyder, T. E., Furberg, C. D., Kowalchuk, G. J., Stuckey, T. D., Rogers, W. J., Givens, D. H., and Waters, D. "Effects of Estrogen Replacement on the Progression of Coronary-Artery Atherosclerosis." *New England Journal of Medicine* 343 (2000): 522–29.

Hulley, S., Furberg, C., Barrett-Connor, E., Cauley, J., Grady, D., Haskell, W., Knopp, R., Lowery, M., Satterfield, S., Schrott, H., Vittinghoff, E., and Hunninghake, D., for the HERS Research Group. "Noncardiovascular Disease Outcomes during 6.8 Years of Hormone Therapy Heart and Estrogen/Progestin Replacement Study Follow-up (HERS II)." *JAMA* 288 (2002): 58–66.

Hulley, S., Grady, D., Bush, T., Furberg, C., Herrington, D., Riggs, B., and Vittinghoff, E. "Randomized Trial of Estrogen Plus Progestin for Secondary Prevention of Coronary Heart Disease in Postmenopausal Women. Heart and Estrogen/Progestin Replacement Study (HERS) Research Group." *JAMA* 280 (1998): 605–13.

Keating, N. L., Cleary, P. D., Rossi, A. S., Zaslavsky, A. M., and Ayanian, J. Z. "Use of Hormone Replacement Therapy by Postmenopausal Women in the United States." *Annals of Internal Medicine* 130 (1999): 545–53.

Lacey, J. V., Mink, P. J., Lubin, J. H., Sherman, M. E., Troisi, R., Hartge, P., Schatzkin, A., and Schairer, C. "Menopausal Hormone Replacement Therapy and Risk of Ovarian Cancer." *JAMA* 288 (2002): 334–41.

LeBlanc, E. S., Janowsky, J., Chan, B. K. X., and Nelson, H. D. "Hormone Replacement Therapy and Cognition: Systematic Review and Meta-Analysis." *JAMA* 295 (2001): 1489–99.

Manson, J. E., and Martin, K. A. "Postmenopausal Hormone-Replacement Therapy." *New England Journal of Medicine* 345 (2001): 34–40.

Mosca, L., Collins, P., Herrington, D. M., Mendelsohn, M. E., Pasternak, R. C., Robertson, R. M., Schenck-Gustafsson, K., Smith, S. C., Taubert, K. A., and Wenger, N. K. "Hormone Replacement Therapy and Cardiovascular Disease: A Statement for Healthcare Professionals from the American Heart Association." *Circulation* 104 (2001): 499–503.

Nelson, H. D., Humphrey, L. L., Nygren, P., Teutsch, S. M., and Allan, J. D. "Postmenopausal Hormone Replacement Therapy." *JAMA* 288 (2002): 872–81.

Rodriguez, C., Patel, A. V., Calle, E. E., Jacob, E. J., and Thun, M. J. "Estrogen Replacement Therapy and Ovarian Cancer Mortality in a Large Prospective Study of US Women." *JAMA* 285 (2001): 1460–65.

Schaumberg, D. A., Buring, J. E., Sullivan, D. A., and Dana, M. R. "Hormone Replacement Therapy and Dry Eye Syndrome." *JAMA* 286 (2001): 2114–19.

Villareal, D. T., Binder, E. F., Williams, D. B., Schechtman, K. B., Yarasheski, K. E., and Kohrt, W. M. "Bone Mineral Density Response to Estrogen Replacement in Frail Elderly Women: A Randomized Controlled Trial." *JAMA* 286 (2001): 815–20.

Worzala, K., Hiller, R., Sperduto, R. D., Mutalik, K., Murabito, J. M., Moskowitz, M., D'Agostino, R. B., and Wilson, P. W. F. "Postmenopausal Estrogen Use, Type of Menopause, and Lens Opacities." *Archives of Internal Medicine* 161 (2001): 1448–54.

Writing Group for the Women's Health Initiative Investigators. "Risks and Benefits of Estrogen Plus Progestin in Healthy Postmenopausal Women." *JAMA* 288 (2002): 321–33.

Growth Hormone

Benbassat, C. A., Maki, K. C., and Unterman, T. G. "Circulating Levels of Insulin-Like Growth Factor (IGF) Binding Protein-1 and -3 in Aging Men: Relationships to Insulin, Glucose, IGF, and Dehydroepiandrosterone Sulfate Levels and Anthropometric Measures." *Journal of Clinical Endocrinology and Metabolism* 82 (1997): 1484–91.

Marcus, R., and Hoffman, A. R. "Growth Hormone as Therapy for Older Men and Women." *Annual Reviews of Pharmacology* 38 (1998): 45–61.

Marcus, R., and Reaven, G. M. "Editorial: Growth Hormone—Ready for Prime Time?" *Journal of Clinical Endocrinology and Metabolism* 82 (1997): 725–26.

Münzer, T., Harman, S. M., Hees, P., Shapiro, E., Christmas, C., Bellantoni, M. F., Stevens, T. E., O'Connor, K. G., Pabst, K. M., St. Clair, C., Sorkin, J. D., and Blackman, M. R. "Effects of GH and/or Sex Steroid Administration on Abdominal Subcutaneous and Visceral Fat in Healthy Aged Women and Men." *Journal of Clinical Endocrinology and Metabolism* 86 (2001): 3604–10.

Rosen, C. J., and Conover, C. "Growth Hormone/Insulin-Like Growth Factor-I Axis in Aging: A Summary of a National Institutes of Aging-Sponsored Symposium." *Journal of Clinical Endocrinology and Metabolism* 82 (1997): 3919–22.

Rudman, D., Feller, A. G., Nagraj, H. S., Gergans, G. A., Lalitha, P. Y., Goldberg, A. F., Schlenker, R. A., Cohn, L., Rudman, I. W., and Mattson, D. E. "Effects of Human Growth Hormone in Men over 60 Years Old." *New England Journal of Medicine* 323 (1990): 1–6.

Vance, M. L., and Mauras, N. "Growth Hormone Therapy in Adults and Children." *New England Journal of Medicine* 341 (1999): 1206–16.

Veldhuis, J. D., Liem, A. Y., South, S., Weltman, A., Weltman, J., Clemmons, D. A., Abbott, R., Mulligan, T., Johnson, M. L., and Pincus, S. "Differential Impact of Age, Sex Steroid Hormones, and Obesity on Basal Versus Pulsatile Growth Hormone Secretion in Men As Assessed in an Ultrasensitive Chemiluminescence Assay." *Journal of Clinical Endocrinology and Metabolism* 80 (1995): 3209–22.

Melatonin

Arendt, J. "Melatonin, Circadian Rhythms, and Sleep." *New England Journal of Medicine* 343 (2000): 1114–16.

Sharkey, K. M., and Eastman, C. I. "Melatonin Phase Shifts Human Circadian Rhythms in a Placebo-Controlled Simulated Night-Work Study." *American Journal of Physiology: Regulatory, Integrative and Comparative Physiology* 282 (2002): R454–R63.

Phytoestrogens

Alekel, D. L., St. Germain, A., Peterson, C. T., Hanson, K. B., Stewart, J. W., and Toda, T. "Isoflavone-Rich Soy Protein Isolate Attenuates Bone Loss in the Lumbar Spine of Perimenopausal Women." *American Journal of Clinical Nutrition* 72 (2000): 844–52.

Burke, G. L., Vitolins, M. Z., and Bland, D. "Soybean Isoflavones As an Alternative to Traditional Hormone Replacement Therapy: Are We There Yet?" *Journal of Nutrition* 130 (2000): 664S–5S.

Busby, M. G., Jeffcoat, A. R., Bloedon, L. T., Koch, M. A., Black, T., Dix, K. J., Heizer, W. D., Thomas, B. F., Hill, J. M., Crowell, J. A., and Zeisel, S. H. "Clinical Characteristics and Pharmokinetics of Purified Soy Isoflavones: Single-Dose Administration to Healthy Men." *American Journal of Clinical Nutrition* 75 (2002): 126–36.

Clarkson, T. B., Anthony, M. S., and Morgan, T. M. "Inhibition of Postmenopausal Atherosclerosis Progression: A Comparison of the Effects of Conjugated Equine Estrogens and Soy Phytoestrogens." *Journal of Clinical Endocrinology and Metabolism* 86 (2001): 41–47.

Davis, S. R. "Phytoestrogen Therapy for Menopausal Symptoms? There's No Good Evidence That It's Any Better than Placebo." *British Medical Journal* 323 (2001): 354–55.

Eden, J. A. "Managing the Menopause: Phyto-Estrogens or Hormone Replacement Therapy?" *Annals of Medicine* 33 (2001): 4–6.

Glazier, M. G., and Bowman, M. A. "A Review of the Evidence for the Use of Phytoestrogens As a Replacement for Traditional Estrogen Replacement Therapy." *Archives of Internal Medicine* 161 (2001): 1161–72.

Gruber, C. J., Tschugguel, W., Schneegerger, C., and Huber, J. C. "Production and Actions of Estrogens." *New England Journal of Medicine* 346 (2002): 340–52.

Kurzer, M. S., and Xu, X. "Dietary Phytoestrogens." *Annual Reviews of Nutrition* 17 (1997): 353–81.

Lichtenstein, A. H. "Got Soy?" *American Journal of Clinical Nutrition* 73 (2001): 667–68.

Nagata, C., Takatsuka, N., Kawakami, N., and Shimizu, H. "Soy Product Intake and Hot Flashes in Japanese Women: Results from a Community-Based Prospective Study." *American Journal of Epidemiology* 153 (2001): 790–93.

Vincent, A., and Fitzpatrick, L. A. "Soy Isoflavones: Are They Useful in Menopause?" *Mayo Clinic Proceedings* 75 (2000): 1174–84.

Raloxifene

Anthony, M., Williams, J. K., and Dunn, B. K. "What Would Be the Properties of an Ideal SERM?" *Annals of the New York Academy of Sciences* 949 (2001): 261–78.

Barrett-Connor, E., Grady, D., Sashegyi, A., Anderson, P. W., Cox, D. A., Hoszowski, K., Rautaharju, P., Harper, K. D., and the MORE Investigators. "Raloxifene and Cardiovascular Events in Osteoporotic Postmenopausal Women. Four-Year Results from the MORE (Multiple Outcomes of Raloxifene Evaluation) Randomized Trial." *JAMA* 287 (2002): 847–57.

Ettinger, B., Black, D. M., Mitlak, B. H., Knickerbocker, R. K., Nickelsen, T., Genant, H. K., Christiansen, C., Delmas, P. D., Zanchetta, J. R., Stakkestad, J., Glüer, C. C., Krueger, K., Cohen, F. J., Eckert, S., Ensrud, K. E., Avioli, L. V., Lips, P., Cummings, S. R., and the Multiple Outcomes of Raloxifene Evaluation (MORE) Investigators. "Reduction of Vertebral Fracture Risk in Postmenopausal Women with Osteoporosis Treated with Raloxifene: Results from a 3-Year Randomized Clinical Trial." *JAMA* 282 (1999): 637–45.

Jordan, V. C., Gapstur, S., and Morrow, M. "Selective Estrogen Receptor Modulation and Reduction in Risk of Breast Cancer, Osteoporosis, and Coronary Heart Disease." *Journal of the National Cancer Institute* 93 (2001): 1449–57.

Lippman, M. E., Krueger, K. A., Eckert, S., Sasegyi, A., Walls, E. L., Jamal, S., Cauley, J. A., and Cummings, S. R. "Indicators of Lifetime Estrogen Exposure: Effect on Breast Cancer Incidence and Interaction with Raloxifene Therapy in the Multiple Outcomes of Raloxifene Evaluation Study Participants." *Journal of Clinical Oncology* 19 (2001): 3111–16.

Mayeux, R. "Can Estrogen or Selective Estrogen-Receptor Modulators Preserve Cognitive Function in Elderly Women?" *New England Journal of Medicine* 344 (2001): 1242–44.

Yaffe, K. "Estrogens, Selective Estrogen Receptor Modulators, and Dementia: What Is the Evidence?" *Annals of the New York Academy of Sciences* 949 (2001): 215–22.

Yaffe, K., Krueger, K., Sarkar, S., Grady, D., Barrett-Connor, E., Cox, D. A., Nickelsen, T., and the Multiple Outcomes of Raloxifene Evaluation Investigators. "Cognitive Function in Postmenopausal Women Treated with Raloxifene." *New England Journal of Medicine* 344 (2001): 1207–13.

Testosterone

Matsumoto, A. M. "Andropause: Clinical Implications of the Decline in Serum Testosterone Levels with Aging in Men." *Journal of Gerontology: Medical Sciences* (2002): M76–M99.

Morley, J. E. "Testosterone Replacement and the Physiologic Aspects of Aging in Men." *Mayo Clinic Proceedings* 75 (2000): S83–S87.

Vermeulen, A. "Androgen Replacement Therapy in the Aging Male—A Critical Evaluation." *Journal of Clinical Endocrinology and Metabolism* 86 (2001): 2380–90.

Chapter 8

General

Chagan, L., Ioselovich, A., Asherova, L., Cheng, J. W. "Use of alternative pharmacotherapy in management of cardiovascular diseases." *American Journal of Managed Care.* 8 (2002):270–85; quiz 286–88, 2002 Mar.

Gillman, M. W., Cupples, L. A., Millen, B. E., Ellison, R. C., and Wolf, P. A. "Inverse Association of Dietary Fat with Development of Ischemic Stroke in Men." *JAMA* 278 (1997): 2145–50.

EDTA

Guldager, B., Jelnes, R., Jorgensen, S. J., Nielsen, J. S., Klaerke, A., Morgensen, K., Larsen, K. E., Reimer, E., Holm, J., and Ottesen, S. "EDTA Treatment of Intermittent Claudication—A Double-Blind, Placebo-Controlled Study." *Journal of Internal Medicine* 231 (1992): 261–67.

L-Carnitine

Barker, G. A., Green, S., Askew, C. D., Green, A. A., and Walker, P. J. "Effect of Propionyl-L-carnitine on Exercise Performance in Peripheral Arterial Disease." *Medicine and Science in Sports and Exercise* 33 (2001): 1415–22.

Benvenga, S., Ruggeri, R. M., Russo, A., Lapa, D., Campenni, A., and Trimarchi, F. "Usefulness of L-carnitine, a Naturally Occurring Peripheral Antagonist of Thyroid Hormone Action, in Iatrogenic Hyperthyroidism: A Randomized, Double-Blind, Placebo-Controlled Clinical Trial." *Journal of Clinical Endocrinology and Metabolism* 86 (2001): 3579–94.

Biagiotti, G., and Cavallini, G. "Acetyl-L-carnitine vs. Tamoxifen in the Oral Therapy of Peyronie's Disease: A Preliminary Report." *BJU International* 88 (2001): 63–67.

Hiatt, W. R., Regensteiner, J. G., Creager, M. A., Hirsch, A. T., Cooke, J. P., Olin, J. W., Gorbunov, G. N., Isner, J., Lukjanov, Y. V., Tsitsiashvili, M. S., Zabelskaya, T. F., and Amato, A. "Propionyl-L-carnitine Improves Exercise Performance and Functional Status in Patients with Claudication." *American Journal of Medicine* 110 (2001): 616–22.

Hurot, J. M., Cucherat, M., Haugh, M., and Fouque, D. "Effects of L-carnitine Supplementation in Maintenance Hemodialysis Patients: A Systematic Review." *Journal of the American Society of Nephrology* 13 (2002): 708–14.

Selimoglu, M. A., Aydogdu, S., Yagci, R. V., and Huseyinov, A. "Plasma and Liver Carnitine Status of Children with Chronic Liver Disease and Cirrhosis." *Pediatrics International* 43 (2001): 391–95.

Wachter, S., Vogt, M., Kreis, R., Boesch, C., Bigler, P., Hoppeler, H., and Krahenbuhl, S. "Long-Term Administration of L-carnitine to Humans: Effect on Skeletal Muscle Carnitine Content and Physical Performance." *Clinica Chimica Acta* 318 (2002): 51–61.

Royal Jelly

Thien, F. C., Leung, R., Baldo, B. A., Weiner, J. A., Plomley, R., and Czarny, D. "Asthma and Anaphylaxis Induced by Royal Jelly." *Clinical and Experimental Allergy* 27 (1997): 1356.

Vittek, J. "Effect of Royal Jelly on Serum Lipids in Experimental Animals and Humans with Atherosclerosis." *Experientia* 51 (1995): 927–35.

Skin

Aizen, E., and Gilhar, A. "Smoking Effect on Skin Wrinkling in the Aged Population." *International Journal of Dermatology* 40 (2001): 431–33.

Fisher, G. J., Wang, Z. Q., Datta, S. C., Varani, J., Kang, W., and Voorhees, J. J. "Pathophysiology of Premature Skin Aging Induced by Ultraviolet Light." *New England Journal of Medicine* 337 (1997): 1419–28.

Gilchrest, B. A. "Aging of the Skin." In: Hazzard, W. R., Blass, J. P., Ettinger, W. H., Halter, J. B., and Ouslander, J. G. *Principles of Geriatric Medicine and Gerontology*. 4th ed. (1999). New York: McGraw-Hill.

Gilchrest, B. A. "A Review of Skin Ageing and Its Medical Therapy." *British Journal of Dermatology* 135 (1996): 867–75.

Additional Resources

Here are some organizations that I recommend for further information:

General

Administration on Aging
www.aoa.gov
(202) 619-0724
330 Independence Avenue SW,
   Washington, D.C. 20201

Agency for Health Care Research
   and Quality
www.ahcpr.gov
(301) 594-1364
2101 East Jefferson Street, Suite 501,
   Rockville, MD 20852

American Cancer Society
www.cancer.org
(800) ACS-2345
1599 Clifton Road NE, Atlanta, GA
   30329

American Dental Association
www.ada.org
(312) 440-2500
211 East Chicago Avenue, Chicago,
   IL 60611

American Diabetes Association
www.diabetes.org
(800) DIABETES
1701 North Beauregard Street,
   Alexandria, VA 22311

American Federation for Aging
   Research
www.afar.org
(212) 703-9977
70 West 40th Street, New York, NY
   10018

American Heart Association
www.americanheart.org
(800) AHA-USA-1
National Center, 7272 Greenville
   Avenue, Dallas, TX 75231

American Lung Association
www.lungusa.org
(212) 315-8700
61 Broadway, Sixth Floor, New York,
   NY 10006

American Medical Association
www.ama-assn.org
(312) 464-5000
515 North State Street, Chicago, IL
   60610

American Public Health Association
www.apha.org
(202) 777-APHA
800 I Street NW, Washington, D.C.
   20001-3710

CDC Diabetes Home Page
www.cdc.gov/diabetes
(877) CDC-DIAB
CDC Division of Diabetes
   Translation, PO Box 8728, Silver
   Spring MD 20910

CDC National Center for Chronic
Disease Prevention and Health
Promotion
www.cdc.gov/nccdphp

Centers for Disease Control and
Prevention
www.cdc.gov
(404) 639-3311
1600 Clifton Road, Atlanta, GA
30333

ClinicalTrials.gov
http://clinicaltrials.gov
(888) FIND-NLM
8600 Rockville Pike, Bethesda, MD
20894

Healthfinder
www.healthfinder.gov
PO Box 1133, Washington, DC
20013-1133

Merriam Webster Medical
Dictionary
www.intelihealth.com/IH/ihtIH/
WSIHW000/9276/9276.html

National Institutes of Health
www.nih.gov
(301) 496-4000
National Institutes of Health,
Bethesda, MD 20892

National Osteoporosis Foundation
www.nof.org
(202) 223-2226
1232 22nd Street NW, Washington,
D.C. 20037-1292

National Stroke Association
www.stroke.org
(800) STROKES
9707 East Easter Lane, Englewood,
CO 80112

NIH National Cancer Institute
www.nci.nih.gov
(800) 4-CANCER
NCI Public Inquiries Office,
Suite 3036A, 6116 Executive
Boulevard, MSC 8322,
Bethesda, MD 20892-8322

NIH National Heart, Lung, and
Blood Institute
www.nhlbi.nih.gov
(301) 592-8573
Building 31, Room 5A52, 31 Center
Drive, MSC 2486, Bethesda, MD
20892

NIH National Institute on Aging
www.nih.gov/nia
(301) 496-1752
Building 31, Room 5C27, 31 Center
Drive, MSC 2292, Bethesda, MD
20892

NIH National Institute on Diabetes
and Digestive and Kidney Diseases
www.niddk.nih.gov
(301) 496-4000
Office of Communications and
Public Liaison, NIDDK, NIH,
Building 31, Room 9A04 Center
Drive, MSC 2560, Bethesda, MD
20892-2560

NIH Senior Health
www.nihseniorhealth.gov

Office of Disease Prevention and
Health Promotion
www.odphp.osophs.dhhs.gov
(202) 205-8611
200 Independence Avenue SW,
Room 738G, Washington, D.C.
20201

Prevent Blindness America
www.preventblindness.org
(800) 331-2020
500 East Remington Road,
    Schaumburg, IL 60173

Robert Wood Johnson Foundation
www.rwjf.org
(888) 631-9989
PO Box 2316, College Road East and
    Route 1, Princeton, NJ 08543

SAMHSA National Clearinghouse
    for Alcohol and Drug
    Information
www.health.org
(800) 729-6686
PO Box 2345, Rockville, MD
    20847-2345

U.S. National Library of Medicine
www.nlm.nih.gov
(888) FIND-NLM
8600 Rockville Pike,
    Bethesda, MD 20894

Nutrition

American Cancer Society
www.cancer.org
(800) ACS-2345
1599 Clifton Road NE,
    Atlanta, GA 30329

American Diabetes Association
www.diabetes.org
(800) DIABETES
1701 North Beauregard Street,
    Alexandria, VA 22311

American Dietetic Association
www.eatright.org
(312) 899-0040
216 West Jackson Boulevard,
    Chicago, IL 60606-6995

American Heart Association
www.americanheart.org
(800) AHA-USA-1
National Center, 7272 Greenville
    Avenue, Dallas, TX 75231

Center for Science in the Public
    Interest
www.cspinet.org
(202) 332-9110
1875 Connecticut Avenue NW,
    Suite 300, Washington, D.C. 20009

FDA Center for Food Safety and
    Applied Nutrition
www.cfsan.fda.gov
(888) SAFEFOOD
5100 Paint Branch Parkway, College
    Park, MD 20740-3835

Food and Drug Administration
    (FDA)
www.fda.gov
(888) INFO-FDA
5600 Fishers Lane, Rockville, MD
    20857-0001

Institute of Medicine, Food and
    Nutrition Board
www.iom.edu
2101 Constitution Avenue NW,
    Washington, D.C. 20418

NIH Clinical Center Nutrition
    Department
www.cc.nih.gov/nutr
10 Center Drive, Bethesda, MD
    20892-1078

National Osteoporosis Foundation
www.nof.org
(202) 223-2226
1232 22nd Street NW, Washington,
    D.C. 20037-1292

Nutrition.Gov
www.nutrition.gov

Tufts Nutrition
http://nutrition.tufts.edu
(617) 636-3736
136 Harrison Avenue,
   Boston, MA 02111

Tufts Nutrition Navigator
www.navigator.tufts.edu

U.S. Department of Agriculture
www.usda.gov
U.S. Department of Agriculture,
   Washington, D.C. 20250

Vegetarian Resource Group
www.vrg.org
(410) 366-8343
PO Box 1463, Baltimore, MD 21203

Exercise

American Alliance for Health,
   Physical Education, Recreation,
   and Dance
www.aahperd.org
(800) 213-7193
1900 Association Drive, Reston, VA
   20191-1598

American Academy of Orthopaedic
   Surgeons
www.aaos.org
(847) 823-7186
6300 North River Road Rosemont,
   Chicago, IL 60018-4262

American College of Sports
   Medicine
www.acsm.org
(317) 637-9200
PO Box 1440,
   Indianapolis, IN 46206-1440

American Council on Exercise
www.acefitness.org
(800) 825-3636
4851 Paramount Drive,
   San Diego, CA 92123

American Heart Association Fitness
   Center
www.justmove.org

CDC National Center for Injury
   Prevention and Control
www.cdc.gov/ncipc
(770) 488-1506
Mailstop K65, 4770 Buford Highway
   NE, Atlanta, GA 30341-3724

President's Council on Physical
   Fitness and Sports
www.fitness.gov
(202) 690-9000
Department W, 200 Independence
   Avenue SW, Room 738-H,
   Washington, D.C. 20201-0004

Weight

Aim for a Healthy Weight (NHLBI)
www.nhlbi.nih.gov/health/public/
   heart/obesity/lose–wt/index.htm

Weight-Control Information Network
   (NIDDK)
www.niddk.nih.gov/health/nutrit/
   win.htm
(877) 946-4627
1 WIN Way, Bethesda, MD 20892-3665

Sleep

American Academy of Sleep Medicine
www.aasmnet.org
(708) 492-0930
One Westbrook Corporate Center,
   Suite 920, Westchester, IL 60154

American Sleep Apnea Association
www.sleepapnea.org
(202) 293-3650
1424 K Street NW, Suite 302,
    Washington, D.C. 20005

National Sleep Foundation
www.sleepfoundation.org
(202) 347-3471
1522 K Street NW, Suite 500,
    Washington, D.C. 20005

NIH National Center on Sleep
    Disorders Research
www.nhlbi.nih.gov/about/ncsdr
(301) 435-0199
Two Rockledge Centre, Suite 10038,
    6701 Rockledge Drive, MSC 7920,
    Bethesda, MD 20892-7920

Engagement

American Psychological Association
www.apa.org
(800) 374-2721
750 First Street NE,
    Washington, DC 20002-4242

National Alliance for the Mentally Ill
www.nami.org
(800) 950-NAMI
Colonial Place Three, 2107 Wilson
    Boulevard, Suite 300, Arlington,
    VA 22201

National Mental Health Association
www.nmha.org
(703) 684-7722
2001 North Beauregard Street,
    12th Floor, Alexandria, VA 22311

NIH National Institute of Mental
    Health
www.nimh.nih.gov
(301) 443-4513
6001 Executive Boulevard,
    Room 8184, MSC 9663,
    Bethesda, MD 20892-8663

Substance Abuse and Mental Health
    Services Administration
www.samhsa.gov
(301) 443-0001
5600 Fishers Lane,
    Rockville, MD 20857

Substance Abuse and Mental Health
    Services Administration's
    Knowledge Exchange Network
www.mentalhealth.org
(800) 789-2647
PO Box 42490, Washington, DC 20015

Shopping

National Institute on Aging, Age
    Page on Health Quackery
www.nia.nih.gov/health/agepages/
    healthqy.htm
(301) 496-1752
National Institute on Aging,
    Building 31, Room 5C27,
    31 Center Drive, MSC 2292,
    Bethesda, MD 20892

U.S. Pharmacopeia
www.usp.org
(800) 227-8772
12601 Twinbrook Parkway,
    Rockville, MD 20852

Index

Boldface page references indicate illustrations. <u>Underscored</u> references indicate boxed text.